Rui Han

Triptolide as a potential aryl hydrocarbon receptor antagonist

Rui Han

Triptolide as a potential aryl hydrocarbon receptor antagonist

Identification of triptolide as a potential aryl hydrocarbon receptor antagonist in human T cells and keratinocytes

Südwestdeutscher Verlag für Hochschulschriften

Impressum/Imprint (nur für Deutschland/only for Germany)
Bibliografische Information der Deutschen Nationalbibliothek: Die Deutsche Nationalbibliothek verzeichnet diese Publikation in der Deutschen Nationalbibliografie; detaillierte bibliografische Daten sind im Internet über http://dnb.d-nb.de abrufbar.

Alle in diesem Buch genannten Marken und Produktnamen unterliegen warenzeichen-, marken- oder patentrechtlichem Schutz bzw. sind Warenzeichen oder eingetragene Warenzeichen der jeweiligen Inhaber. Die Wiedergabe von Marken, Produktnamen, Gebrauchsnamen, Handelsnamen, Warenbezeichnungen u.s.w. in diesem Werk berechtigt auch ohne besondere Kennzeichnung nicht zu der Annahme, dass solche Namen im Sinne der Warenzeichen- und Markenschutzgesetzgebung als frei zu betrachten wären und daher von jedermann benutzt werden dürften.

Coverbild: www.ingimage.com

Verlag: Südwestdeutscher Verlag für Hochschulschriften GmbH & Co. KG
Heinrich-Böcking-Str. 6-8, 66121 Saarbrücken, Deutschland
Telefon +49 681 37 20 271-1, Telefax +49 681 37 20 271-0
Email: info@svh-verlag.de

Approved by: Kiel, CAU, 2011

Herstellung in Deutschland (siehe letzte Seite)
ISBN: 978-3-8381-3213-6

Imprint (only for USA, GB)
Bibliographic information published by the Deutsche Nationalbibliothek: The Deutsche Nationalbibliothek lists this publication in the Deutsche Nationalbibliografie; detailed bibliographic data are available in the Internet at http://dnb.d-nb.de.

Any brand names and product names mentioned in this book are subject to trademark, brand or patent protection and are trademarks or registered trademarks of their respective holders. The use of brand names, product names, common names, trade names, product descriptions etc. even without a particular marking in this works is in no way to be construed to mean that such names may be regarded as unrestricted in respect of trademark and brand protection legislation and could thus be used by anyone.

Cover image: www.ingimage.com

Publisher: Südwestdeutscher Verlag für Hochschulschriften GmbH & Co. KG
Heinrich-Böcking-Str. 6-8, 66121 Saarbrücken, Germany
Phone +49 681 37 20 271-1, Fax +49 681 37 20 271-0
Email: info@svh-verlag.de

Printed in the U.S.A.
Printed in the U.K. by (see last page)
ISBN: 978-3-8381-3213-6

Copyright © 2012 by the author and Südwestdeutscher Verlag für Hochschulschriften GmbH & Co. KG and licensors
All rights reserved. Saarbrücken 2012

Aus der Klinik für Dermatologie, Venerologie und Allergologie
(Direktor: Prof. Dr. med. Thomas Schwarz)
im Universitätsklinikum Schleswig-Holstein, Campus Kiel
an der Christian-Albrechts-Universität zu Kiel

IDENTIFICATION OF TRIPTOLIDE AS A POTENTIAL ARYL HYDROCARBON RECEPTOR ANTAGONIST IN HUMAN T CELLS AND KERATINOCYTES

Inauguraldissertation
zur
Erlangung der Doktorwürde
der Medizinischen Fakultät
der Christian-Albrechts-Universität zu Kiel
vorgelegt von

RUI HAN

aus Shandong, Volksrepublik China

Kiel 2011

List of abbreviations

AhR	Aryl hydrocarbon receptor
CYP1A1	Cytochrome P450 1A1
CYP1B1	Cytochrome P450 1B1
DMSO	Dimethylsulfoxide
DTNB	5,5-dithiobis-2-nitrobenzoic acid
EC	Effective concentration
EDTA	Ethylene diamine tetra acetate
ELISA	Enzyme-linked immunosorbent assay
FACS	Fluorescent activated cell sorting
FICZ	6-formylindolo[3,2-b]carbazole
HRQoL	Health-related quality of life
MTT	3-(4,5-Dimethylthiazol-2-yl)-2,5-diphenyltetrazolium bromide
NF-kB	Nuclear factor kappa B
NHEK	Normal human epidermal keratinocytes
NR	Neutral red
PBMCs	Peripheral blood mononuclear cells
PBS	Phosphate buffered saline
PGE2	prostaglandin E2
TCDD	2,3,7,8-tetra-chlorodibenzo-p-dioxin
TP	Triptolide
Treg	Regulatory T cells
XRE	Xenobiotic responsive element

Index

1. Introduction .... - 6 -
   1.1 Background .... - 6 -
   1.2 Purpose of the study .... - 11 -
   2.1 Cell culture .... - 12 -
      2.1.1 Cell lines .... - 12 -
         2.1.1.1 Normal human epidermal keratinocytes (NHEK) .... - 12 -
         2.1.1.2 Naïve T cells .... - 12 -
            2.1.1.2.1 Human peripheral blood mononuclear cells (PBMCs) isolation .... - 12 -
            2.1.1.2.2 Naïve T cells separation .... - 12 -
      2.1.2 Cell culture conditions .... - 13 -
   2.2 Neutral red assay .... - 14 -
      2.2.1 Principles of neutral red assay .... - 14 -
      2.2.2 Procedures of neutral red assay .... - 14 -
   2.3 MTT assay .... - 15 -
      2.3.1 Principles of MTT assay .... - 15 -
      2.3.2 Procedures of MTT assay .... - 16 -
   2.4 Quantitative Real-time Reverse transcriptase (RT)-PCR assays ...... - 16 -
      2.4.1 Treatment of cells with FICZ and TP .... - 16 -
      2.4.2 RNA isolation .... - 17 -
      2.4.3 Formaldehyde Denaturing Agarose Gel Electrophoresis of RNA - 17 -
         2.4.3.1 Principle of Formaldehyde Denaturing Agarose Gel Electrophoresis .... - 17 -
         2.4.3.2 Procedure of Formaldehyde Denaturing Agarose Gel Electrophoresis .... - 18 -
            2.4.3.2.1 Preparation of buffer and gel .... - 18 -
            2.4.3.2.2 Preparation of RNA samples .... - 18 -
            2.4.3.2.3 Electrophoresis .... - 18 -
      2.4.4 Reverse transcription .... - 19 -
      2.4.5 Real time quantitative PCR and data analysis .... - 19 -
   2.5 Fluorescent Activated Cell Sorting (FACS) analysis .... - 20 -

- **2.5.1 Principle of flow cytometric analysis** .... - 20 -
- **2.5.2 Procedure of FACS analysis** .... - 20 -
  - 2.5.2.1 Treatment of cells with FICZ and TP .... - 20 -
  - 2.5.2.2 Cell stimulation .... - 21 -
  - 2.5.2.3 Staining of the cells with antibodies .... - 21 -
    - 2.5.2.3.1 Surface staining with antibody against CD45-PE .... - 21 -
    - 2.5.2.3.2 Intracellular staining with antibodies against IL-17, IL-22 and IFN-γ .... - 21 -
  - 2.5.2.4 Flow cytometric analysis .... - 22 -
- **2.6 Apo2.7 cytotoxicity test in Naïve T cells** .... - 22 -
  - **2.6.1 Principles of Apo2.7 assay** .... - 22 -
  - **2.6.2 Procedures of Apo2.7 assay** .... - 22 -
    - 2.6.2.1 Treatment of cells with TP .... - 22 -
    - 2.6.2.2 Cell stimulation .... - 23 -
    - 2.6.2.3 Staining of the cells with antibodies .... - 23 -
      - 2.6.2.3.1 Surface staining with antibody against CD45-PE .... - 23 -
      - 2.6.2.3.2 Intracellular staining with antibodies against Apo 2.7 .. - 23 -
    - 2.6.2.4 Flow cytometric analysis .... - 24 -
- **2.7 Enzyme-linked immunosorbent assay (ELISA)** .... - 24 -
  - **2.7.1 Principle of ELISA** .... - 24 -
  - **2.7.2 Procedure of ELISA** .... - 24 -
    - 2.7.2.1 Treatment of cells with FICZ and TP .... - 24 -
    - 2.7.2.3 IL-17A, IL-22 and IFN-γ detection with ELISA .... - 25 -
- **2.8 Statistical analysis** .... - 26 -
- **3. Results** .... - 27 -
  - **3.1 Neutral red assay** .... - 27 -
  - **3.2 MTT assay** .... - 28 -
  - **3.3 Quantitative Real-time RT-PCR assays** .... - 30 -
    - 3.3.1 Formaldehyde Denaturing Agarose Gel Electrophoresis of RNA - 30 -
    - 3.3.2 Expression of mRNA of CYP1A1 and CYP1B1 in NHEK .... - 31 -
    - 3.3.3 Expression of mRNA of IFN-γ, IL-17, IL-22, CYP1A1 and CYP1B1 in naïve T cells .... - 32 -
  - **3.4 FACS analysis** .... - 33 -
  - **3.5 Apo2.7 cytotoxicity test in naïve T cells** .... - 40 -

3.6 ELISA	- 42 -
4. Discussion	- 44 -
5. Summary	- 48 -
6. Reference	50
7. Acknowledgements	61
8. Curriculum Vitae	62

1. Introduction

1.1 Background

Psoriasis is an immune-mediated inflammatory disease of the skin affecting 2-3% of the Caucasian and 0.123% of the Chinese population (Raychaudhuri and Farber, 2001;Yip, 1984). It is characterized by sharply demarcated erythematous plaques with silvery scales which appear typically on the knees, elbows, sacral region and scalp, but the entire skin may be involved. The pathogenesis of psoriasis is still not fully understood. A genetic predisposition and immunologic mechanisms seem to be mainly responsible for the development of skin lesions (Lowes et al., 2007). Psoriasis negatively affects patients' health-related quality of life (HRQoL) and results in a significant socioeconomic burden.

Treatment of psoriasis is related to the extent of lesions and recent guidelines on evidence-medicine based criteria provide helpful background information on the choice of different drugs or regimens (Nast et al., 2007). Whereas in mild psoriasis according to a recent definition topical therapy is recommended systemic therapy is indicated for moderate to severe psoriasis (Mrowietz, 2011). There is the choice between conventional therapies such as methotrexate, ciclosporin and fumaric acid esters as first-line and biologic agents as second-line systemic treatment.

Recent data on the pathogenesis of psoriasis focus on the involvement of specifically activated T cells on the background of a genetic susceptibility with HLA-Cw6 being the most important susceptibility gene. It is well known that dysregulated or uncontrolled effector T cell responses can lead to autoimmune diseases. $CD4^+$ T cells expand and differentiate into different effector cells termed Th1, Th2, Th17 and Tregs characterized by the production of a certain subset of cytokines (Bettelli et al., 2007;Mucida et al., 2007). The induction and progression of many autoimmune diseases is thought to be mediated by Th1 cells (Chang et al., 1997;Raychaudhuri and Farber, 2001). Identification of the Th17 family of effector T cells represented a major recent breakthrough (Kolls and Linden, 2004;Yao et al., 1995). Besides IL-17A, Th17 cells also release IL-17F, IL-21 and IL-22 (Korn et al., 2007;Liang et al., 2006;Nurieva et al., 2007). It is currently believed that Th17 cells play a central role in host defense against certain pathogens and an exaggerated Th17 response might lead to autoimmune diseases and severe inflammatory responses (Cooper,

2007;Kolls and Linden, 2004). Th17 differentiation is regulated by various cytokines. Th17 differentiation can be induced by TGF-β and IL-6 in mice, and is further enhanced by IL-1β and IL-21 in humans (Bettelli, Korn, and Kuchroo, 2007;Stockinger et al., 2007). The development of Th17 cells is negatively regulated by IFN-γ and IL-27, the signals of which are dependent on STAT1, and IL-2, dependent on STAT5, respectively (Harrington et al., 2005;Laurence et al., 2007;Stumhofer et al., 2006). In addition to cytokines, other mediators may impact Th17 cells differentiation. It has been shown that prostaglandin E2 (PGE2) favors human Th17 expansion (Boniface et al., 2009;Chizzolini et al., 2008;Napolitani et al., 2009). More recently, two groups have reported that the activated aryl hydrocarbon receptor (AhR) regulates regulatory T cells (Treg) and Th17 cell development and promotes Th17 polarization (Quintana et al., 2008;Veldhoen et al., 2008).

AhR, also known as dioxin receptor, is a ubiquitous ligand-activated basic helix-loop-helix-PAS (bHLH-PAS)-44-containing transcription factor present in the cytoplasm. AhR binds to and is activated by a range of structurally divergent chemicals including natural dietary, endogenous ligands, and synthetic environmental agents among which dioxin (2,3,7,8-tetra-chlorodibenzo-p-dioxin (TCDD)) is the most extensively studied pure agonist (Beischlag et al., 2008;Bradshaw and Bell, 2009;Nebert and Karp, 2008). Upon binding with a ligand, AhR undergoes a conformation change, translocates to the nucleus, and dimerizes with AhR nuclear translocator (Arnt). It regulates the expression of a variety of genes, including the xenobiotic metabolizing enzyme cytochrome P450 1A1 (CYP1A1) and cytochrome P450 1B1 (CYP1B1) (Denison and Nagy, 2003). Interestingly, it has been recently reported that AhR is a ligand-dependent E3 ubiquitin ligase (Ohtake et al., 2007), implying that AhR has dual functions in controlling intracellular protein levels, serving both as a transcriptional factor to promote the induction of target proteins and as a ligand-dependent E3 ubiquitin ligase to regulate selective protein degradation.

There is considerable evidence to suggest that AhR signaling plays a role in the function of the immune system. A substantial amount of literature (Okey, 2007) described interactions of AhR with other key regulatory proteins including NF-κB (Tian et al., 2002), which has a role in immune-mediated inflammation such as psoriasis. The nuclear AhR complex binds to the core nucleotide sequence xenobiotic responsive element (XRE), which occurs frequently in the mammalian genome and is also represented in IL-17A, IL-17F, IL-22 and ROR-γt. It has been demonstrated that agonists of the AhR play an integral role in T cell function, promoting a Th2/Th1 switch resulting in a Th1 bias (Negishi et al., 2005). In the CD4$^+$ T-cell lineage of mice AhR expression is restricted to the Th17 cell subset and its ligation results in the production of the Th17 cytokine IL-22. AhR-deficient mice showed decreased IL-17 development and absence of IL-22 production (Veldhoen et al., 2008). Th17 differentiation of mice naive CD4+ T cells was markedly inhibited in the presence of the AhR antagonist CH-223191. Additionally, it was shown that AhR was only induced under Th17-cell-inducing conditions. Collectively, Th17 differentiation represents an alternative biological system in which the effects of potential AhR agonists or antagonists can be directly tested.

A number of compounds are described as AhR antagonists, including the flavone derivatives α-napthoflavone (α-NF) (Wilhelmsson et al., 1994), 5´-methoxy-6´-aminoflavone (PD98059) (Reiners, Jr. et al., 1998) and 3´-methoxy-4´-nitroflavone (MNF) (Lu et al., 1995), 6-methoxy-1,3,8-trichlorodibenzofuran (6-MCDF) (Astroff et al., 1988;Harris et al., 1989), 1-amino-3, 7, 8-trichlorodibenzo-p-dioxin (Luster et al., 1986), omeprazole sulphide (Gerbal-Chaloin et al., 2006) and 6, 2´, 4´-trimethoxyflavone (TMF) (Murray et al., 2010). Interestingly, the plant kingdom is rich in AhR ligands predominantly in the form of polyphenolic flavonoid compounds. Many of these compounds exhibit anti-oxidant, anti-proliferative and anti-inflammatory activities.

Extracts of the herb Tripterygium wilfordii Hook F. (TwHF), also known as "Lei Gong Teng", are used as one of the most common systemic treatments for diseases such as psoriasis in China mainly due to its favourable cost-benefit ratio. TwHF has been used for centuries in traditional Chinese medicine to treat rheumatoid arthritis. Originally, an extract obtained by boiling TwHF in water (decoction) was used for systemic treatment. Since a number of adverse effects were observed during therapy the extraction method was changed (Tao and Lipsky, 2000). With the aim to reduce toxicity an ethyl acetate extract and a chloroform–methanol extract (T2) were developed in the 1970s (Gutian Hospital and Beisha Hospital, 1972). Both of these preparations are commercially available in China and have been used extensively meanwhile.

The extracts of TwHF contain more than 70 ingredients including diterpenoids, triterpenoids, sesquiterpenoids, β-sitosterol, dulcitol, and glycosides (Chen, 2001). Triptolide ($C_{20}H_{24}O_6$, chemical structure see Figure 1) turned out to be the active substance of TwHF extracts, which has been shown to possess potent anti-inflammatory and immunosuppressive properties *in vitro* as well as in different animal models in numerous preclinical studies (Asano et al., 1998;Chang, Chang, Kuo, and Chang, 1997;Chang et al., 1993;Ho et al., 1999;Tao et al., 1998). Beside its use for the treatment of psoriasis, it has been shown that triptolide inhibits experimental autoimmune uveoretinitis and prolongs allograft survival (Kupchan et al., 1972;Wu et al., 2003a). Moreover, it has been demonstrated that a succinyl derivative of triptolide, PG490-88, can prevent graft-versus-host disease (Chen et al., 2002). In addition to the anti-inflammatory and immunosuppressive activities, triptolide also exhibits potent anti-tumor and anti-leukemic activities (Jiang et al., 2001;Liu et al., 2004;Wang et al., 2006).

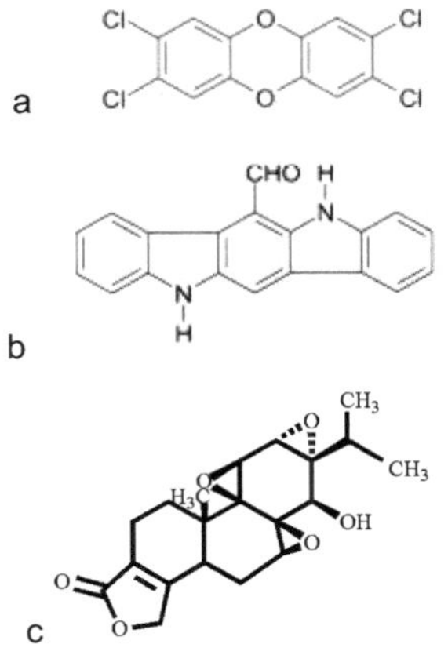

Figure 1. Chemical structure of TCDD (a), FICZ (b) and triptolide (c).

The immunosuppressive action of triptolide has been generally attributed to suppression of T-lymphocyte activation. Triptolide induces apoptosis in lymphocytes and decreases the expression of IL-2 and IFN-γ in T cells by inhibiting nuclear factor-kB (NF-kB) translocation (Chan et al., 1999;Qiu and Kao, 2003).
In mice triptolide acts on the tumour necrosis factor α (TNFα)/tumour necrosis factor receptor 2 pathway of lymphocytes in the colon inhibiting the activation of NF-κB as well as the expression of IFN-γ (Wei et al., 2008). Furthermore, triptolide inhibits the production of IL-3, 4, 5, 6, and 8 by lymphocytes (Qiu and Kao, 2003). Recently, it was found that triptolide inhibited the differentiation of murine CD4[+] T cells into Th17 cells in a dose dependent manner (Wang et al., 2008a). Triptolide decreased the

transcription level of IL-17 mRNA and IL-6-induced phosphorylation of STAT3, a key signaling molecule involved in the development of Th17 cells.

1.2 Purpose of the study

From the molecular structure of triptolide (Figure 1) the hypothesis was generated that the compound could bind to AhR and serve as either agonist or antagonist. For this purpose it was investigated whether triptolide could induce cell death and affect FICZ induced CYP1A1 and CYP1B1 transcription on human keratinocytes. It was further explored if the exposure to triptolide could affect differentiation of naïve human T cells to Th17 cells and FICZ induced IFN-γ, IL-17, IL-22, CYP1A1 and CYP1B1 transcription on naïve human T cells.

2 Materials and Methods
2.1 Cell culture
2.1.1 Cell lines
2.1.1.1 Normal human epidermal keratinocytes (NHEK)

Primary NHEK were purchased from Promocell (Heidelberg, Germany). NHEK-c adult were derived from adult normal human tissue from different locations, e.g. face, breast, abdomen, and thighs. Primary NHEK were cryopreserved in 1ml serum-free freezing medium (Cryo-SFM, PromoCell) in liquid nitrogen, containing >500 000 viable cells after thawing.

2.1.1.2 Naïve T cells

2.1.1.2.1 Human peripheral blood mononuclear cells (PBMCs) isolation

Human peripheral blood was collected in micro-hematocrit capillary tubes (Sarstedt, Nümbrecht, Germany) with 1mM ethylene diaminetetraacetic acid (EDTA) and diluted with the same volume of Dulbecco's phosphate-buffered saline (PBS, without Ca & Mg, PAA Laboratories, Pasching, Austria). The dilution was underlayered by density gradient centrifugation using Ficoll-Paque separation medium (PAA Laboratories), and centrifuged for 30 min at 400 ×g at 18°C. The interphase containing mononuclear cells was harvested and washed twice with cold (6-8°C) PBS. The pellet was resuspended in 5ml ACK Lysis Buffer, which was prepared with 0.15M NH_4Cl, 10mM $KHCO_3$ and 0.1mM EDTA (all from Merck, Darmstadt, Germany) in ddH_2O and adjusted to PH 7.2-7.4. The cell suspension was incubated at room temperature for 5 minutes with occasional shaking. The reaction was stopped by diluting the Lysis Buffer with 30ml PBS and the cells were spinned at 400 ×g at 4°C. The number of cells was evaluated by staining with 0.4% trypan blue (Sigma-Aldrich, Steinheim, Germamy) and counting using a Bürker chamber.

2.1.1.2.2 Naïve T cells separation

2.1.1.2.2.1 Principle of the MACS® (Miltenyi Biotec) Separation

Using the Naïve CD4+ T Cell Isolation Kit II (Miltenyi Biotech, Bergisch Gladbach, Germany), human untouched naïve $CD4^+$ $CD45RA^+$ T cells are isolated by depletion of non-T helper cells and memory $CD4^+$ T cells. Non-T helper cells and memory $CD4^+$ T cells are indirectly magnetically labeled with a cocktail of biotin-conjugated monoclonal antibodies, as primary labeling reagent, and Anti-Biotin MicroBeads, as secondary labeling reagent. The magnetically labeled non-T helper cells and memory

CD4⁺ T cells are depleted by retaining them on a MACS® Column in the magnetic field of a MACS Separator (both from Miltenyi Biotech), while the unlabeled naive CD4⁺ T cells pass through the column.

2.1.1.2.2.2 Procedure of the MACS® Separation

MACS buffer was prepared containing PBS, 0.5% bovine serum albumin (BSA, Sigma-Aldrich), and 2 mM EDTA, filtered through 0.2 µm pore membrane (Sarstedt), and stored at 4°C. The cells were spinned at 300 ×g at 4°C and the pellet was resuspended in 40 µl of MACS buffer per 10^7 total cells. 10 µl of Naive CD4⁺ T Cell Biotin-Antibody Cocktail II per 10^7 total cells was added and well mixed. The cells were incubated for 10 minutes at 4°C and washed by adding 2 ml of buffer per 10^7 cells and centrifuging at 300×g for 10 minutes. The supernatant was aspirated completely and the cell pellet was resuspended in 80 µl of buffer per 10^7 total cells. 20 µl of Anti-Biotin MicroBeads per 10^7 total cells was added and well mixed. Thereafter the cells were incubated for 15 minutes at 4°C, washed repeatedly and resuspended in 500 µl of buffer.

LS column was placed in the magnetic field of MACS Separator, and rinsed with 3ml buffer. The cell suspension was applied onto the column and flow-through containing unlabeled cells was collected in collection tube. The column was washed three times with the 3ml buffer and the total effluent was collected and combined with the effluent before, which comprised the enriched naive CD4⁺CD45RA⁺ T cell fraction. The cells were spinned at 400 ×g at 4°C. The number of cells was evaluated by staining with 0.4% trypan blue and counting using a Bürker chamber.

2.1.2 Cell culture conditions

NHEK of passage 2 were re-cultured in serum-free keratinocyte growth medium 2 (PromoCell) supplemented freshly with SupplementMix (PromoCell) at 37°C in a 5% CO_2 atmosphere. NHEK was passaged by dissociation in trypsin/EDTA solution (0.04% trypsin/0.03% EDTA, PromoCell) for NHEK and trypsin neutralizing solution (0.05% trypsin inhibitor with 0.1% BSA, PromoCell). NHEK of passage 4 were used for the experiments.

Naïve T cells were resuspended in RPMI (Gibco BRL, Karlsruhe, Germany) supplemented with 10% fetal calf serum (FCS , PAA Laboratories), HEPES (10 mM, Sigma-Aldrich), penicillin (100 U/ml), streptomycin (100 µg/ml, Biochrom AG, Berlin) and L-glutamine (2 mM, Biochrom AG, Berlin) in 24-well flat bottom plates (Sarstedt), and stimulated with plate-bound anti-CD3 mAb (clone OKT3, 2.5 µg/ml) and anti-CD28 mAb (clone 28.2, 1 µg/ml, BioLegend, San Diego, USA). For human Th17 differentiation, cells were supplemented with 10 ng/ml recombinant IL-1β and 20 ng/ml recombinant IL-6, 10 ng/ml IL-23 (all from R&D Systems, Wiesbaden, Germany), 1 ng/ml recombinant human transforming growth factor-beta (TGF-β, CHO cell-derived, PromoCell), as previously reported.

2.2 Neutral red assay

2.2.1 Principles of neutral red assay

The neutral red assay was developed for the assessment of the effect of toxic agents on cells in culture. The assay is based on the incorporation of the supravital dye neutral red (NR) into the lysosomes of viable cells after their incubation with toxic chemicals. This weakly cationic dye penetrates cell membranes by nonionic diffusion and binds intracellularly to sites of the lysosomal matrix (Lüllmann-Rauch, 1979). Xenobiotics that injure the plasma or lysosomal membrane decrease the uptake and subsequent retention of the dye. Dead or damaged cells cannot retain the dye after the washing and fixation procedures. After NR has been extracted from the lysosomes, it can be quantitated spectrophotometrically and the amount compared with the amount of dye extracted from control cell cultures. Quantification of the extracted dye has been shown to be linear with cell numbers (Borenfreund and Puerner, 1985a;Borenfreund and Puerner, 1985b).

2.2.2 Procedures of neutral red assay

Individual wells of a 96-well tissue culture microtiter plate were seeded with 0.2 ml of normal NHEK culture medium containing 2×10^4 NHEK cells, to achieve a 70 to 80% confluence after attachment and one day incubation. After 24h of incubation, the media were removed and replaced with 0.2 ml control medium or with 0.2ml medium with various concentrations of triptolide (TP, Sigma-Aldrich), which ranged from 0.05µM, 0.1µM, 0.25µM to 0.5µM with a concentration of the primary solvent DMSO (Sigma-Aldrich) of 0.2%. Naïve T cells were seeded at a density of 2×10^5 /ml per well in the 96-well plates, treated with different concentration TP (0.3µM, 0.1µM, 0.06µM, 0.03µM, 0.01µM, 0.003µM, 0.0003µM) respectively and incubated in a humidified atmosphere with 5% CO_2 at 37°C, in supplemented RPMI medium for 24 hours. Cells cultured in only medium served as control.

After 24h of exposure to TP the media were removed and replaced with 0.1ml/well medium containing 100µg of NR (Sigma-Aldrich) per ml (except for negative control). The NR-containing media were pre-incubated overnight at room temperature and filtered (0.2µm) prior to use to remove fine precipitates of dye crystals. The assay plate was then returned to the incubator for another 3 h to allow for uptake of the supravital dye into the lysosomes of viable cells. Thereafter, the media were removed and the cells were rapidly washed with 0.2 ml/well 1% formaldehyde-1% $CaCl_2$ (all from Fluka, Buchs, Switzerland) followed by 0.2 ml/well of a solution of 1% acetic acid (Merck)-50% ethanol (J.T. Baker, Deventer, Netherlands) to extract the dye from the cells. After 10 min at room temperature and a brief but rapid agitation on a microtiter plate shaker, the plates were transferred to a microplate reader (SunriseTM Remote, TECAN, Austria) equipped with a 540-nm filter to measure the absorbance of the extracted dye at 540-nm versus 405-nm. The EC25 was calculated as the concentration of the agent (TP) at which 25% of the cells were positive for NR.

2.3 MTT assay

2.3.1 Principles of MTT assay
Yellow MTT (3-(4,5-Dimethylthiazol-2-yl)-2,5-diphenyltetrazolium bromide, a tetrazole) is reduced to purple formazan in the mitochondria of living cells. The absorbance of this colored solution can be quantified by measuring at a certain wavelength (usually between 500 and 600 nm) by a spectrophotometer. The absorption max is dependent on the solvent employed. This reduction takes place only when mitochondrial reducing enzymes are active and therefore conversion can be directly related to the number of viable (living) cells. When the amount of purple formazan produced by cells treated with an agent is compared with the amount of formazan produced by untreated control cells, the effectiveness of the agent in causing death of cells can be deduced, through the production of a dose-response curve. Solutions of MTT solubilized in tissue culture media or balanced salt solutions, without phenol red, are yellowish in color. Mitochondrial dehydrogenases of viable cells cleave the tetrazolium ring, yielding purple MTT formazan crystals which are insoluble in aqueous solutions. The crystals can be dissolved in acidified isopropanol. The resulting purple solution is spectrophotometrically measured. An increase in cell number results in an increase in the amount of MTT formazan formed and an increase in absorbance. The MTT

method of cell determination is useful in the measurement of cell growth in response to mitogens, antigenic stimuli, growth factors and other cell growth promoting reagents, cytotoxicity studies, and in the derivation of cell growth curves (Michael et al., 1988;SLATER et al., 1963;van de Loosdrecht et al., 1940).

2.3.2 Procedures of MTT assay

For the experiments MTT (Sigma-Aldrich) was freshly prepared as 5 mg/ml in PBS without phenol red and serum, filtered (0.2 μm) prior to use and kept for 5 min at 37°C. Individual wells of a 96-well tissue culture microtiter plate were seeded with 0.2 ml of normal NHEK culture medium containing 2×10^4 NHEK cells, to achieve a 70 to 80% confluence after attachment and one day incubation. After 24h of incubation, the medium was removed and replaced with 0.2ml control medium or with 0.2ml medium with various concentrations of TP, which ranged from 0.003μM, 0.01μM,0.03μM,0.05μM,0.08μM, 0.1μM, to 0.16μM with a concentration of the primary solvent DMSO (Sigma-Aldrich) of 0.2%. Naïve T cells were seeded at a density of 2×10^5 /ml per well in the 96-well plates, treated with different concentration TP (0.3μM, 0.1μM, 0.06μM, 0.03μM, 0.01μM, 0.003μM, 0.0003μM) respectively and incubated in a humidified atmosphere with 5% CO_2 at 37°C, in supplemented RPMI medium for 24 hours. Cells cultured in only medium served as control.

After 24h of exposure to TP, the media were removed by aspiration and replaced with 0.1ml/well medium containing 20μl MTT solution. The assay plate was then returned to the incubator for another 4 h to allow for uptake of MTT into the mitochondria of viable cells. Thereafter, the media were removed and replaced by 0.15 ml/well of a solution of 0.1% Nondet P-40 (NP40) with 4 mM HCl in isopropanol to dissolve the resulting purple MTT formazan crystals. The plate was then incubated in 37°C with agitation on a microtiter plate shaker to enhance dissolution. After 15 min, the plate was transferred to a microplate reader (Sunrise^{TM} Remote) equipped with a 570 nm filter to measure the absorbance of the extracted dye at 570 nm versus 690 nm.

2.4 Quantitative Real-time Reverse transcriptase (RT)-PCR assays
2.4.1 Treatment of cells with FICZ and TP

2×10^5 NHEK were seeded to 24-well plates and cultured in normal NHEK medium to achieve about 80% ~90% confluence after attachment and 24-hour incubation. After washing with warm PBS once, cells were treated with 0.05μM FICZ, 0.05μM TP or 0.05μM FICZ with different concentration TP (0.05μM, 0.025μM, 0.001μM) respectively in 1ml supplemented RPMI medium and incubated in a humidified atmosphere with 5% CO_2 at 37°C for 24 hours. Cells cultured in only medium served as control.

Naïve T cells were seeded at a density of 2×10^6 /ml per well in the 24-well plates, treated with 0.03μM FICZ, 0.03μM TP or 0.03μM FICZ with different concentration TP (0.03μM, 0.003μM, 0.0003μM) respectively and incubated in a humidified atmosphere with 5% CO_2 at 37°C, in supplemented RPMI medium for 24 hours. Cells cultured in only medium served as control.

2.4.2 RNA isolation

Total RNA from NHEK or naïve T cells were extracted using Trizol reagent, according to the manufacturer's instruction (Invitrogen, Karlsruhe, Germany). At the end of incubation, medium was removed. Cells were lysed by adding 0.5 ml per well of Trizol reagent and homogenized for 5 minutes at room temperature to permit the complete dissociation of nucleoprotein complexes. Each sample was mixed with 100μl chloroform (Sigma-Aldrich) at room temperature for 10 minutes. After centrifugation at 8800×g for 15 minutes at 4°C, the supernatants were mixed with 250μl 70% isopropanol (J.T.Baker) and kept at -20°C overnight. RNA pellets were collected by centrifugation at 8800×g for 10 minutes at 4°C. After washing with 0.5 ml 75% ethanol (J.T.Baker), pellets were dissolved in 20 μl water. Aliquots of RNA were stored at -80°C until further use.

2.4.3 Formaldehyde Denaturing Agarose Gel Electrophoresis of RNA

2.4.3.1 Principle of Formaldehyde Denaturing Agarose Gel Electrophoresis

Denaturing agarose gel electrophoresis is used to control the size and integrity of RNA preparations. RNA has the tendency to form both secondary and tertiary structures that can impede its separation by electrophoresis. As such, identical species of RNA exhibiting varying degrees of intra molecular base pairing migrate at different rates and result in the smearing of distinct RNA molecules. Consequently, the electrophoresis of RNA needs to be performed under denaturing conditions. Heat denaturing the RNA sample prior to electrophoresis is insufficient, as secondary structures will simply reform unless a denaturing system is used. Successful electrophoresis of RNA is therefore accomplished in two steps: RNA is heat denatured prior to electrophoresis; during electrophoresis conditions have been established maintaining the RNA in a denatured state.

In this assay, both formaldehyde and formamide are added to the sample before electrophoresis to aid the denaturation of the RNA sample (Sambrook, 1989).

2.4.3.2 Procedure of Formaldehyde Denaturing Agarose Gel Electrophoresis

2.4.3.2.1 Preparation of buffer and gel

10×MOPS buffer was prepared with 200 mM 3-[N-morpholino]propanesulfonic acid (MOPS, free acid, Sigma-Aldrich), 50 mM sodium acetate and 10 mM EDTA in ddH_2O, and adjusted to pH 7.0 with NaOH.

A Formaldehyde Agarose gel (1.2 % agarose) of size 10×14×0.7 cm was prepared using a mixture of 1.2 g agarose, 10 ml 10x MOPS buffer and RNase-free water to a final volume of 100 ml. The mixture was heated briefly to melt agarose and cooled to 65°C in a water bath. 1.8 ml of 37% (12.3 M) formaldehyde (Fluka) and 10 µl SYBR® Green II RNA gel stain (10,000×concentrate in DMSO, Invitrogen) was added, mixed thoroughly and poured onto gel support with a comb that will form wells large enough to accommodate at least 25 µl.

Formaldehyde Agarose gel running buffer was prepared with 20 ml 10x MOPS buffer, 4 ml 37% (12.3 M) formaldehyde and 176 ml RNase-free water.

The gel was assembled in the tank after 30 min, and covered by a few millimeters with 1× Formaldehyde Agarose gel running buffer. The comb was then removed, and the gel was equilibrated in 1x Formaldehyde Agarose gel running buffer for at least 30 min.

2.4.3.2.2 Preparation of RNA samples

5x loading buffer was prepared with 16 µl saturated aqueous bromophenol blue solution, 80 µl 500 mM EDTA, 720 µl 37% (12.3 M) formaldehyde, 2 ml 100% glycerol (Sigma-Aldrich), 3084 µl formamide, 4 ml 10 x MOPS buffer and RNase-free water to a final volume of 10 ml. 16µl of RNA sample containing 1µg RNA was mixed with 4µl of 5x loading buffer and incubated for 10 min at 65°C.

2.4.3.2.3 Electrophoresis

The denatured RNA was chilled on ice and loaded onto the equilibrated formaldehyde agarose gel. To avoid overheating and a smile effect on the migration of RNA and staining dye the gel was run at 5–7 V/cm in 1x formaldehyde agarose gel running buffer until the SYBR Green II dye has moved approximately half to three quarters of the way along the gel. RNA was visualized using a 300-nm short-wave ultraviolet transilluminator. Pictures of gels were taken at f 4.5 for 1/2-1s.

2.4.4 Reverse transcription

RNA concentration (µg/µl) was determined by measuring the optical density at 260 nm with RNA/DNA calculator software Gene Quant. Equal amounts of total RNA from each sample were reverse-transcribed into cDNA with standard reagents according to the recommendations of the manufacturer (Invitrogen). 1 µg RNA was incubated with 0.75µg oligo (dT) 18 primer (Fermentas, Mainz, Germany) for 10 minutes at 70°C. After incubation RNA was transferred into a reaction mixture containing 4µl 5×first-strand buffer (250 mM Tris-HCl, pH 8.3 at room temperature; 375 mM KCl; 15 mM $MgCl_2$), 2µ1 DTT (100 mM), 1µl dNTPs (10 mM), and 0.25µl Superscript II^{TM} reverse transcriptase (all from Invitrogen) and incubated at 42°C for 60 minutes. Transcription was stopped at 90°C for 5 minutes. Thereafter the products were stored at -80°C until further use.

2.4.5 Real time quantitative PCR and data analysis

Real time quantitative PCR and data analysis was carried out using pre-developed QuantiTect primer assays for human IFN-γ (Hs00989291_m1), IL-17 (Hs00174383_m1), IL-22 (Hs001574154_m1), CYP1A1 (Hs00153120_m1), CYP1B1 (Hs009164383_m1) and GapdH (Hs99999905_m1, all from Applied Biosystem, New Jersey, USA) with FAM detection on an ABI Prism 7300 Sequence Detection System (Roche Diagnostics, Manheim, Germany).

cDNA corresponding to 25 ng RNA served as a template in a 20 µl reaction system containing 0.9 µM of each primer and 1×TaqMan Universal PCR Master Mix (Applied Biosystem). Samples were loaded into MicroAmp® Optical 96-Well Reaction Plate (Applied Biosystem) and sealed with adhesive covers (Applied Biosystem). The plates were centrifuged briefly to remove air bubbles and collect the liquid at the bottom, and then incubated in the thermal cycler block for an initial activation of AmpliTaq Gold enzyme at 95°C for 30 seconds followed by 45 cycles, each cycle consisting of denaturing by 95°C for 15 seconds and extending by 60°C for 1 min.

In all cases, melting point analysis revealed amplification of a single product. Data acquisition and analysis were achieved using Applied Biosystem software (Applied Biosystem). Relative abundance of each target transcript in unstimulated or stimulated samples was normalized to GapdH using the formula $2^{-\Delta CT}$, where $\Delta Ct = Ct^{TARGET} - Ct^{GapdH}$. Fold change values correspond to the difference of target transcript relative abundance in stimulated compared to unstimulated samples and were calculated using the formula $2^{-\Delta\Delta CT}$, where $\Delta\Delta Ct = \Delta Ct^{STIMULATED} - \Delta Ct^{UNSTIMULATED}$.

2.5 Fluorescent Activated Cell Sorting (FACS) analysis
2.5.1 Principle of flow cytometric analysis

Flow cytometry is the measurement of various physicochemical characteristics of suspended cells. The procedure is typically performed in combination with the use of fluorescent probes that stain cellular components or functions (Shapiro, 2005). Using a microfluidic system that directs a high-speed single-file stream of cells to a focused laser beam in a glass capillary tube, flow cytometers capture light scattering at different angles and fluorescence emissions at several wavelengths for each individual cell. Detected light signals are collected by a series of optical systems and processed by data-analysis electronics to measure morphological, biochemical and functional properties of cells such as size, shape, DNA content, cell surface markers, cell cycle distribution and viability. Such combined implementation of microfluidics, optics and electronics in modern flow cytometers provides a robust platform to quantify multiple characteristics of sample populations (e.g. cells, viruses, bacteria, yeast, aerosol particles, microbeads) simultaneously at high rates (up to approximately 25000 cells/s). For the past three decades, advances in precision technologies, dye synthesis and high-speed data-handling techniques have exerted synergistic effects on flow cytometry, bringing this powerful analytical tool into routine clinical and laboratory use in the field of cell/molecular biology (Boeck, 2001), disease diagnostics (Stein et al., 1992), immunology (Gabriel and Kindermann, 1995), genetics (Wedemeyer and Potter, 2001) and environmental monitoring (Dubelaar and Gerritzen, 2000).

2.5.2 Procedure of FACS analysis
2.5.2.1 Treatment of cells with FICZ and TP

Naïve T cells were seeded at a density of 1×10^6 /ml per well in the 24-well plates with plate-bound anti-CD3 mAb (clone OKT3, 2.5 µg/ml) and anti-CD28 mAb (clone 28.2, 1 µg/ml) in supplemented RPMI medium. For human Th17 differentiation, cells were supplemented with 10 ng/mL recombinant IL-1β and 20 ng/ml recombinant IL-6, 100 ng/ml IL-23, 1 ng/ml TGF-β, as previously reported.

The cells were treated from the beginning with 0.5µM FICZ, 0.5µM FICZ plus different concentration of TP or left with supplemented medium alone respectively and incubated in a humidified atmosphere with 5% CO_2 at 37°C for 72 hours. TP was added to the wells at final concentrations of 0.03µM, 0.003µM and 0.0003µM per well.

2.5.2.2 Cell stimulation

After 72-hours incubation periods, the cells of every well were transferred into a 1.5 ml sterile centrifuge tube (Sarstedt) and washed twice with PBS. Cells were resuspended in 200µl RPMI medium and pipetted to 96-well U-bottom plate (Sarstedt). PdBU 50 nM, Ionomycin 500 ng/ml and Brefaldin A 10 µg/ml was added to each well. The plate was incubated with 5% CO_2 at 37°C for three hours.

2.5.2.3 Staining of the cells with antibodies

2.5.2.3.1 Surface staining with antibody against CD45-PE

FACS buffer was prepared with 2% heat inactivated FCS and 0.09% (w/v) sodium azide in Dulbecco's PBS , adjusted to pH 7.4-7.6, filtered through 0.2 µm pore membrane, and stored at 4°C. Cells after 3h incubation were washed once with FACS buffer by centrifugation at 400×g at 4°C for 5 minutes. Thereafter, cells were pre-incubated with 5ul mouse serum for 10 min at room temperature to block non-specific binding. Then cells were resuspended in 50ul FACS buffer with 5µl fluorochrome-conjugated monoclonal antibody CD45-PE or the corresponding PE-labeled immunoglobulin isotype control antibody as control and incubated for 20 min at 4°C in dark. Thereafter cells were washed twice with 150µl/well FACS buffer and supernatant was discarded.

2.5.2.3.2 Intracellular staining with antibodies against IL-17, IL-22 and IFN-γ

Cells were thoroughly resuspended in 200 µl of BD Cytofix/Cytoperm™ solution for 20 min at room temperature. Then all wells were washed two times in 1×BD Perm/Wash™ solution. The fixed/permeabilized cells were thoroughly resuspended in 50 µl of BD Perm/Wash™ solution, containing 5ul Anti-IL17-Pc5.5 Conjugated Antibody (clone eBio64DEC17, ebioscience) , 5ul Anti-IL22-PE Conjugated Antibody (clone BG/IL22, BioLegend) and 5ul Anti- IFN-γ-PE-Cy7 Conjugated Antibody (clone 4S.B3, ebioscience) or corresponding IgG1-Pc5.5,IgG1-PE and IgG1-PECy7 -labeled isotype control antibodies as control. After 30 min incubation at 4°C in the dark, cells were washed two times with FACS buffer to remove all unbound reagents and resuspended in 500µl FACS Buffer prior to flow cytometric analysis.

2.5.2.4 Flow cytometric analysis

Analysis was performed using an EPICS-XL flow cytometer together with system II software (Beckman-Coulter). Cells were gated according to forward and side scatter characteristics. For each sample, at least of 100 000 viable cells were analyzed and the results were expressed as the mean percentage of cells staining positive.

2.6 Apo2.7 cytotoxicity test in naïve T cells
2.6.1 Principles of Apo2.7 assay

Apoptosis, or programmed cell death, plays a fundamental role in many normal biological processes as well as several disease states (Cohen et al., 1992;Ellis et al., 1991;Nicholson, 1996;Thompson, 1995;Wyllie et al., 1980). Apoptosis can be induced by various stimuli that all produce the same end result: systematic and deliberate cell death. The 2.7A6A3 monoclonal antibody (mAb) reacts with the APO2.7 antigen (also called 7A6 antigen) that is a 38 kDa mitochondrial membrane protein which appears to be exposed on cells undergoing apoptosis (programmed cell death). It has been suggested that APO2.7 protein is involved in the molecular cascade of apoptosis and its expression represents an early event of apoptosis rather than a final product of dead cells (Zhang et al., 1996). Normal viable cells are negative or weakly positive for APO2.7. Research studies have shown that less than 2% of peripheral T cells from normal donors expressed the APO2.7 antigen. Some level of APO2.7 expression associated with an on-going apoptotic process has been demonstrated in activated T cells. By flow cytometric analysis, the APO2.7 antigen can be detected after apoptosis induction via CD95/Fas ligation, irradiation or drug treatment. The 2.7A6A3 mAb strongly reacts with cells induced to undergo apoptosis (Pepper et al., 1998;Zhang et al., 1996). In contrast, this mAb fails to stain or weakly stains untreated and digitonin-permeabilized human peripheral blood cells and hematopoietic cell lines (Jurkat, Molt-4, etc.). Apo2.7 also reacts specifically with apoptotic Jurkat cells induced by gamma-irradiation, Ara-C treatment, or CD95 (Fas) antibody ligation (Koester et al., 1997;Zhang et al., 1996).

2.6.2 Procedures of Apo2.7 assay
2.6.2.1 Treatment of cells with TP

For determination of Apo2.7-expression, naïve T cells were seeded at a density of 1×10^6/ml per well in the 24-well plates, respectively and incubated in a humidified atmosphere with 5% CO_2 at 37°C, in supplemented RPMI medium for 24 hours. The cells were treated from the beginning with TP or left with supplemented RPMI medium alone. TP was added to the wells at final concentrations of 0.3µM, 0.1µM, 0.06µM, 0.03µM and 0.01µM per well. Cells without any addition of TP served as a medium control.

2.6.2.2 Cell stimulation

After 24-hours incubation periods, the cells of every well was transferred into a 1.5 ml sterile centrifuge tube (Sarstedt) and washed twice with PBS. Cells were resuspended in 200µl RPMI medium and pipetted to 96-well U-bottom plate. Phorbol-12-13-dibutyrate (PdBU) 50 nM, Ionomycin 500 ng/ml and Brefaldin A 10 µg / ml was added to each well. The plate was incubated with 5% CO_2 at 37°C for three hours.

2.6.2.3 Staining of the cells with antibodies
2.6.2.3.1 Surface staining with antibody against CD45-PE

Cells after 3h incubation were washed once with FACS buffer by centrifugation at 400 ×g at 4°C for 5 minutes. Thereafter, cells were pre-incubated with 5ul mouse serum (eBioscience) for 10 min at room temperature to block non-specific binding. Then cells were suspended in 50ul FACS buffer with 5µl fluorochrome-conjugated monoclonal antibody CD45-PE (Beckman coulter, Marseille, France) or the corresponding PE-labeled immunoglobulin isotype control antibody as control. The cell suspension was incubated for 20 min at 4°C in dark. Thereafter cells were washed twice with 150µl/well FACS buffer and supernatant was removed.

2.6.2.3.2 Intracellular staining with antibodies against Apo 2.7

Cells were thoroughly resuspended in 200 µl of BD Cytofix/Cytoperm™ (BD bioscience, San Diego, CA, USA) solution for 20 min at room temperature. Then all wells were washed two times in 1×BD Perm/Wash™ solution. The fixed/permeabilized cells were thoroughly resuspended in 50 µl of BD Perm/Wash™ solution, containing 5ul Anti-APO2.7-Pc5 Conjugated Antibody (clone 2.7A6A3, Beckman-Coulter, Krefeld) or corresponding PC5-labeled isotype control antibodies (DAKO, Glostrup, Denmark) as control. After 30 min incubation at 4°C in the dark, cells were washed two times with FACS buffer to remove all unbound reagents and resuspended in 500μl FACS Buffer prior to flow cytometric analysis.

2.6.2.4 Flow cytometric analysis

The apoptosis-inducing effect of TP on Naïve T cells was assessed by single colour flow cytometry. Analysis was performed using an EPICS-XL flow-cytometer together with system II software (Beckman-Coulter). Cells were gated according to forward and side scatter characteristics. For each sample, at least of 100 000 viable cells were analyzed and the results were expressed as the mean percentage of cells staining positive. Experiments were performed in duplicate.

2.7 Enzyme-linked immunosorbent assay (ELISA)
2.7.1 Principle of ELISA

ELISA is a rapid immunochemical test that involves an enzyme (a protein that catalyzes a biochemical reaction). It also involves an antibody or antigen (immunologic molecules). ELISA tests are utilized to detect substances that have antigenic properties, primarily proteins (as opposed to small molecules and ions such as glucose and potassium). It is a highly sensitive and specific method in estimating ng/ml to pg/ml ordered materials in the solution, such as serum, urine, sperm and culture supernatant (Savige et al., 1998).

There are variations of this test, but the most basic consists of an antibody attached to a solid surface. This antibody has affinity for (will latch on to) the substance of interest, for example, human chorionic gonadotropin (HCG), the commonly measured protein which indicates pregnancy. A mixture of purified HCG linked (coupled) to an enzyme and the test sample (blood, urine, etc) are added to the test system. If no HCG is present in the test sample, then only HCG with linked enzyme will bind. The more HCG which is present in the test sample, the less enzyme linked HCG will bind. The substance the enzyme acts on is then added, and the amount of product measured in some way, such as a change in color of the solution.

2.7.2 Procedure of ELISA
2.7.2.1 Treatment of cells with FICZ and TP

Naïve T cells were seeded at a density of 1×10^6/ml per well in the 24-well plates with plate-bound anti-CD3 mAb (clone OKT3, 2.5 μg/ml) and anti-CD28 mAb (clone 37.51, 1 μg/ml) in supplemented RPMI medium. For human Th17 differentiation, cells were

supplemented with 10 ng/ml recombinant IL-1β and 20 ng/ml recombinant IL-6, 10 ng/ml IL-23, 1 ng/ml TGF-β, as previously reported.
The cells were treated from the beginning with 0.5μM FICZ, 0.5μM FICZ plus different concentration of TP or left with supplemented medium alone respectively and incubated in a humidified atmosphere with 5% CO_2 at 37°C for 72 hours. TP was added to the wells at final concentrations of 0.03μM, 0.01μM and 0.003μM per well.

2.7.2.2 Cell stimulation

After 72-hours incubation period, the cells of each well were transferred into a 1.5 ml sterile centrifuge tube and washed twice with PBS. Cells were resuspended in 200μl RPMI medium and pipette to 96-well plate. PdBU 50 nM and ionomycin 500 ng/ml was added to each well. The plate was incubated at 37°C in a 5% CO_2 atmosphere. After five hours, cells were spinned and the supernatants were stored in new 1.5ml sterile centrifuge tube in -80°C for ELISA.

2.7.2.3 IL-17A, IL-22 and IFN-γ detection with ELISA

The ELISA was carried out according to the manufacturer's instruction of Human IL-17A ELISA Ready-SET-Go!™ Kit, Human IL-22ELISA Ready-SET-Go!™ Kit and Human IFN-γ ELISA Ready-SET-Go!™ Kit (all from eBioscience). The high affinity protein binding plates (Corning Costar 9018) were pre-coated with 100 μl/well of IL-17, IL-22 or IFN-γ capture antibody in coating Buffer (1:250 diluted) respectively, sealed with mylar and incubated overnight at 4°C. Each plate was washed 5 times with 250 μl/well wash buffer (0.05% Tween-20 in PBS) the next day. Thereafter the wells were blocked with 200 μl/well of 1×Assay Diluent and incubated at room temperature for 1 hour. After five times washing, 100 μl/well of individual standard dilution (diluted with 1×Assay Diluent to concentrations of 7.8125 pg/μl, 15.625 pg/μl, 31.25 pg/μl, 62.5 pg/μl, 125 pg/μl, 250 pg/μl and 500 pg/μl) and sample dilutions (1:10 diluted with 1×Assay Diluent) were added to the appropriate wells. The plates were sealed and incubated overnight at 4°C for maximal sensitivity. After a repetition of washing steps the next day, 100 μl/well of IL-17, IL-22 or IFN-γ detection antibody (1:250 diluted in 1×Assay Diluent) was added to respective plates. Then the plates were sealed and incubated at room temperature for one hour. 100 μl/well of Avidin Horseradish Peroxidase (AV-HRP, 1:250 diluted in 1×Assay Diluent) was added after repeated washing steps. The plates were sealed and incubated at room temperature for 30 min. Then 100 μl/well of Tetramethylbenzidine (TMB) substrate solution was added to each well after seven times aspirate and wash of the plates. The addition of 50 μl of stop solution (1M H_3PO_4) is completed into the wells. The plate was transferred to a microplate reader (Sunrise™ Remote) within 30 minutes and the absorbance was measured with a 450 nm filter. A formula made according to the concentration and respective ΔOD/min of standards was used to quantify samples measured.

2.8 Statistical analysis

The data obtained in our study were expressed as mean ± standard deviation. EC values and corresponding 95% confidence intervals were calculated by SPSS software (SPSS, Inc., USA). Statistical significance between groups of the samples was evaluated by t-test. A *p*-value below 0.05 was considered significant and indicated by one asterisk (*), and *p*-value below 0.01 was considered significant and indicated by two asterisk (**).

3. Results

3.1 Neutral red assay

TP-induced cytotoxicity in keratinocytes was determined by using the neutral red assay. NHEK were cultured with TP for 24h. The following concentrations of TP were used: 0.05µM, 0.1µM, 0.25µM and 0.5µM. After 24h incubation with TP a small proportion of the cultured cells were found dead as observed under the inverted microscope. The proportion of damaged cells differed according to the different TP-concentrations. The relative neutral red absorbance corresponding to different TP-concentrations is shown in Figure 2. Generally, absorbance of neutral red increased when the TP concentration decreased. The EC_{25} value of TP in NHEK could be calculated as 0.0547µM. Therefore, 0.05µM was used as the highest concentration of TP in the following experiments with NHEK.

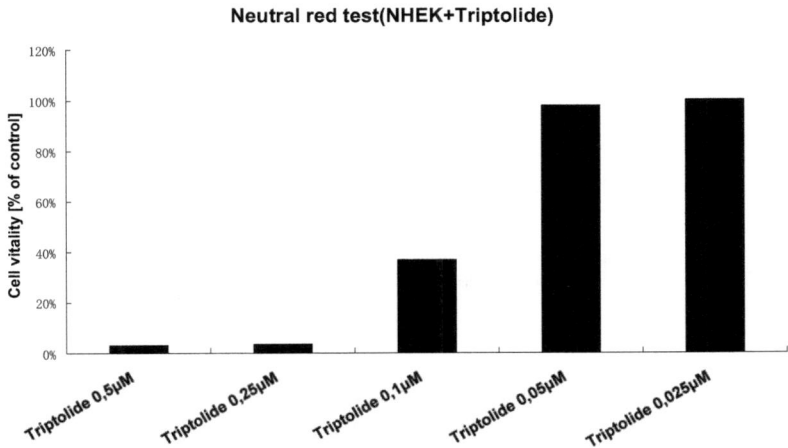

Figure 2 Relative absorbance of neutral red corresponding to different TP concentrations in NHEK. Mean of two independent experiments.

To detect cytotoxicity effects of TP in naïve T cells, the following concentrations of TP were used: 0. 30µM, 0.10µM, 0.06µM, 0.03µM, 0.01µM, 0.003µM and 0.0003µM.

After 24h incubation with TP a small proportion of the cultured cells were found dead as observed under the inverted microscope. The proportion of damaged cells differed according to the different TP-concentrations. The relative neutral red absorbance corresponding to different TP-concentrations is shown in Figure 3.The EC_{25} value of TP in Naïve T cells could be calculated as 0.0282µM. Therefore, 0.03µM was used as the highest concentration of TP in the following experiments with Naïve T cells.

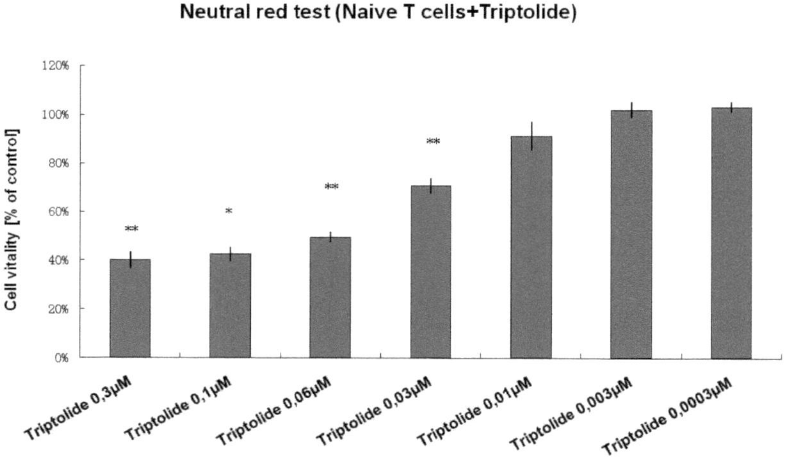
Neutral red test (Naive T cells+Triptolide)
Cell vitality [% of control]
120%
100%
80%
60%
40%
20%
0%
**
*
**
**
Triptolide 0,3µM
Triptolide 0,1µM
Triptolide 0,06µM
Triptolide 0,03µM
Triptolide 0,01µM
Triptolide 0,003µM
Triptolide 0,0003µM

Figure 3 Relative absorbance of neutral red corresponding to different TP concentrations in Naïve T cells. Mean ± SD of four independent experiments. ***P*<0.01;**P*<0.05.

3.2 MTT assay

To detect effects of TP on the proliferation of keratinocytes, NHEK were incubated with different concentrations of TP (0. 16, 0.10, 0.08, 0.05, 0.03, 0.01, 0.003µM) or 0.16µM FICZ. Cells were harvested for MTT analysis after 24h-incubation. The relative MTT absorbance corresponding to different TP concentrations is shown in Figure 4. Absorbance of MTT increased when the TP concentration decreased. TP at concentrations above 0.03µM showed a significant inhibitory effect on the proliferation of keratinocytes (*P*<0.01). FICZ showed no inhibitory effect at the concentration of

0.16µM.

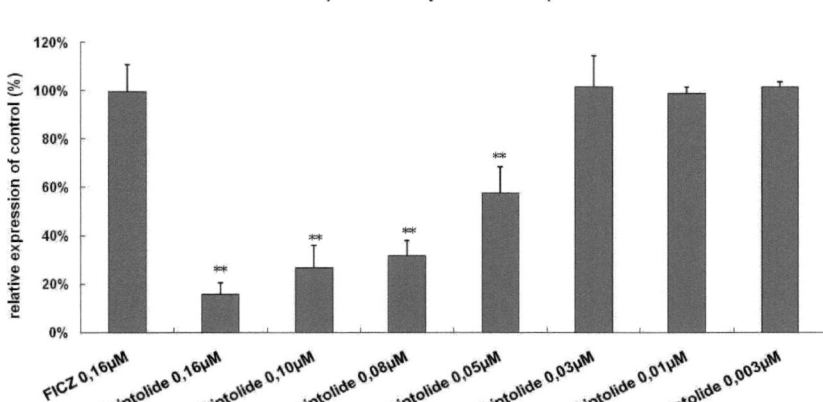

Figure 4 TP inhibited proliferation of keratinocytes in a dose-dependent fashion. Mean ± SD of three independent experiments. **$P<0.01$.

To detect effects of TP on the proliferation of naïve T cells, the following concentrations of TP was used: 0. 30, 0.10, 0.06, 0.03, 0.01, 0.003, 0.0003µM. Cells were harvested for MTT analysis after 24h-incubation. The relative MTT absorbance corresponding to different TP concentrations is shown in Figure 5. Absorbance of MTT increased when the TP concentration decreased. TP at concentrations above 0.003µM showed a significant inhibitory effect on the proliferation of keratinocytes ($P<0.05$).

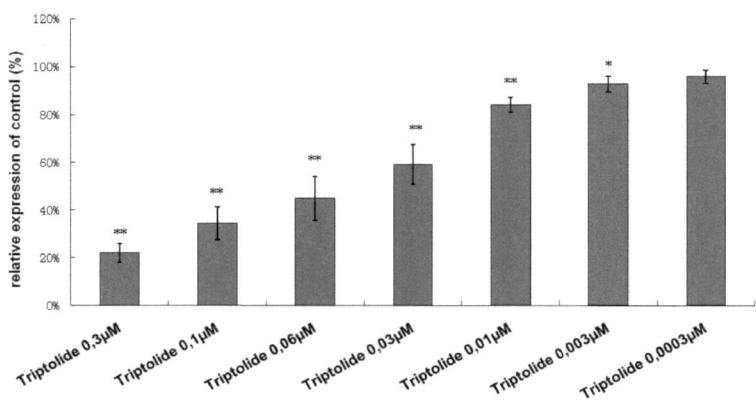

Figure 5 TP inhibited proliferation of naïve T cells in a dose-dependent fashion. Mean ± SD of four independent experiments. $**P<0.01; *P<0.05$.

3.3 Quantitative Real-time RT-PCR assays

3.3.1 Formaldehyde Denaturing Agarose Gel Electrophoresis of RNA

To assess the quality of RNA after cell lysis, denaturing agarose gel electrophoresis was performed before quantitative real-time PCR. One μg of degraded total RNA from each sample was subjected to a 1.2% denaturing agarose gel and visualized on a UV transilluminator. Intact total RNA on a denaturing gel showed sharp 28S and 18S rRNA bands (eukaryotic samples). The 28S rRNA band was approximately twice as intense as the 18S rRNA band (Figure 6). This 2:1 ratio (28S:18S) was a good indicator for RNA integrity. These RNA-preparations were used for further quantitative real-time PCR.

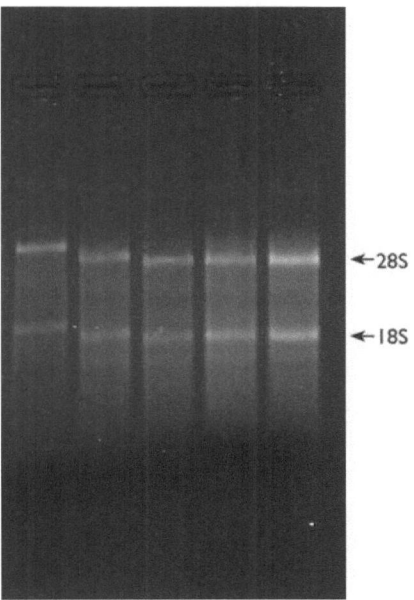

Figure 6 Formaldehyde denaturing agarose gel electrophoresis of RNA. The 18S and 28S ribosomal RNA bands are clearly visible in the intact RNA sample.

3.3.2 Expression of mRNA for CYP1A1 and CYP1B1 in NHEK

To examine the effect of TP on AhR-responsive transcriptor production at mRNA levels, quantitative real-time PCR was used to determine the level of CYP1A1 and CYP1B1 mRNA expression in human keratinocytes. NHEK (2×10^5) were incubated with FICZ (0.05µM) alone or FICZ (0.05µM) and different concentrations of TP (0.05µM, 0.025µM, 0.001µM). Total RNA was harvested after 24h-incubation and the expression of CYP1A1 and CYP1B1 was determined by quantitative real-time PCR analysis. Data represent relative mRNA levels of the indicated target gene normalized against Hprt. As shown in figure 7 FICZ-induced AhR-dependent CYP1A1 and CYP1B1 expression was significantly inhibited by TP at a concentration of 0.05µM in NHEK.

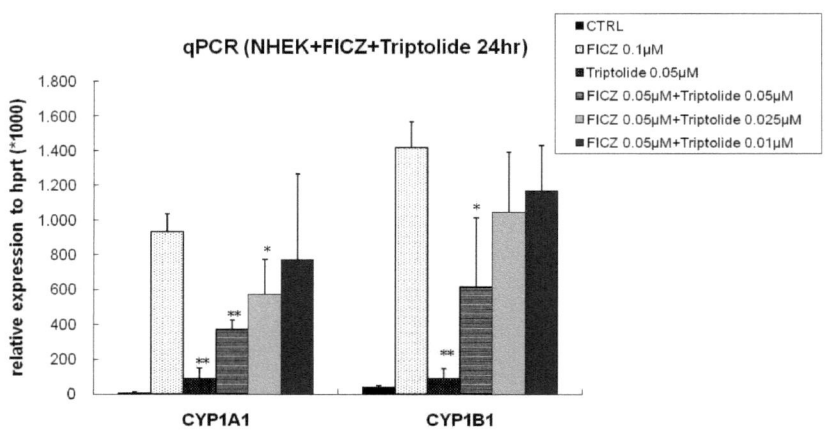

Figure 7 Inhibitory effect of TP on FICZ-induced production of CYP1A1 and CYP1B1 by NHEK at the transcriptional level. Mean + SD of at least three independent experiments. **$P<0.01$.* $P<0.05$.

3.3.3 Expression of mRNA of IFN-γ, IL-17, IL-22, CYP1A1 and CYP1B1 in naïve T cells

Naïve T cells (2×10^6) were incubated with FICZ (0.03μM) alone or FICZ (0.03μM) together with TP (0.03μM, 0.003μM, 0.0003μM). Total RNA was harvested after 24h-incubation and FICZ-induced AhR-dependent mRNA-expression of CYP1A1 and CYP1B1, IFN-γ, IL-17 and IL-22 was determined by quantitative real-time PCR analysis. Data shown in figure 8 represent relative mRNA levels of the indicated target gene normalized against GAPDH. FICZ-induced expression of AhR-dependent CYP1A1, CYP1B1, IFN-γ, IL-17 and IL-22 was significantly inhibited by TP at a concentration of 0.03μM in naïve T cells.

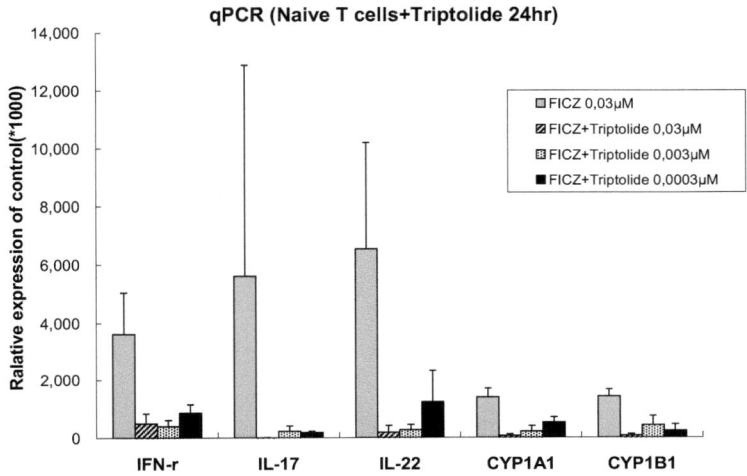

Figure 8 Inhibitory effect of TP on FICZ-induced mRNA-expression of CYP1A1, CYP1B1, IFN-γ, IL-17 and IL-22 in naïve T cells. Mean + SD of three independent experiments. **$P<0.01$.* $P<0.05$.

3.4 FACS analysis

To determine the effect of TP on the intracellular expression of cytokines by naïve T cells, 1×10^6 naïve T cells were incubated with FICZ (0.03μM) alone or with FICZ (0.03μM) and TP (0.03μM, 0.003μM, 0.0003μM). Cells were restimulated with PDBU, ionomycin and brefaldin A after 72h-incubation. Cells were washed, incubated with fluorescence labeled antibodies and analyzed at the single cell level by FACS. The results showed that there are very few IL-17- and IL-22-producing T cells in control cultures stimulated with anti-CD3 and anti-CD28 mAb (Figure 9). Addition of IL-1β, IL-6, IL-23 and TGF-β promoted the expression of IL-22 and IL-17 (Figure 10) in particular together with the addition of FICZ (Figure 11). In this experimental setting TP inhibited IL-17-, IL-22- and IFN-γ-expression as shown in Figures 12, 13 and 14. In the presence of 0.03μM TP only one division of cells (IFN-γ) was observed (Figure 12) suggesting that TP could inhibit the division in IL-1β/IL-6/IL-23/ TGF-β antibody-stimulated naïve T cells. The inhibition of cytokines showed a significant dose-related effect as compared to the FICZ-induced cultures (Figure 15). The data was representative of three independent experiments with similar results.

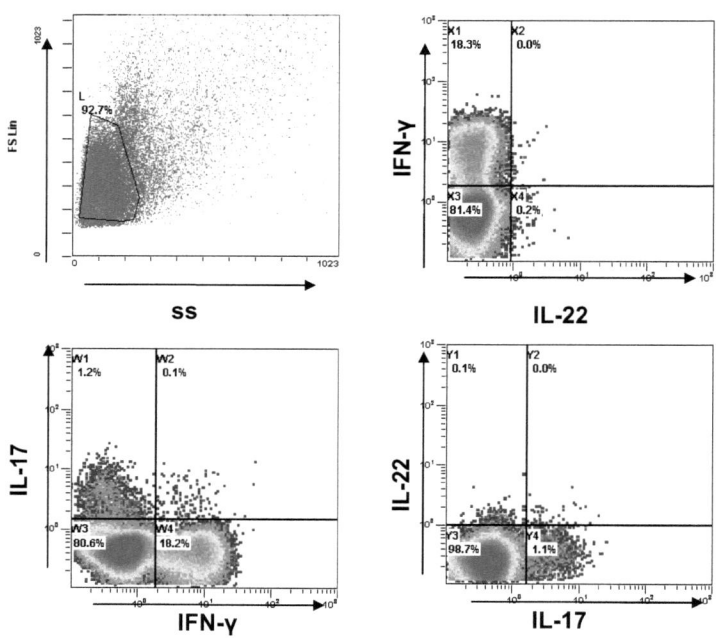

Figure 9 Flow cytometric analysis of IFN-γ, IL-17 and IL-22 in T cells stimulated with anti-CD3 and anti-CD28 mAb.

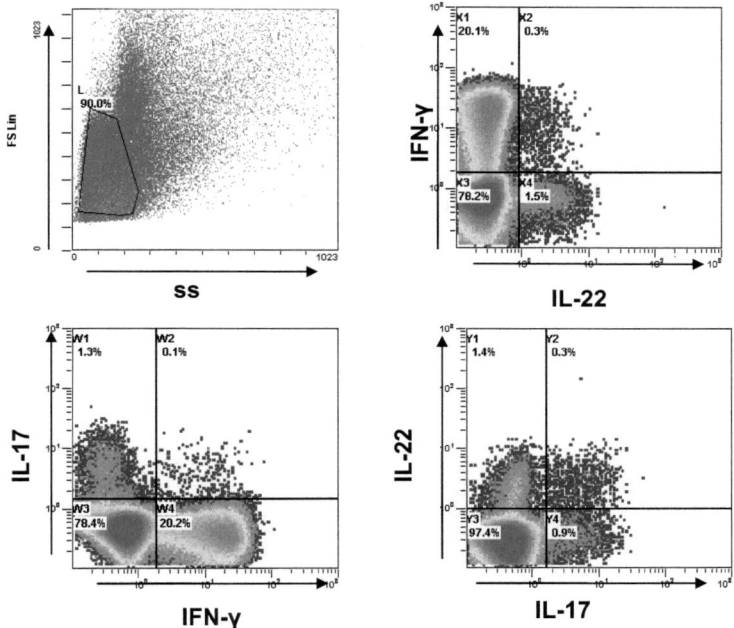

Figure 10 Flow cytometric analysis of IFN-γ, IL-17 and IL-22 in T cells stimulated with 10 ng/ml IL-1β, 20 ng/ml IL-6, 10 ng/ml IL-23, 1 ng/ml TGF-β together with anti-CD3 and anti-CD28 mAb.

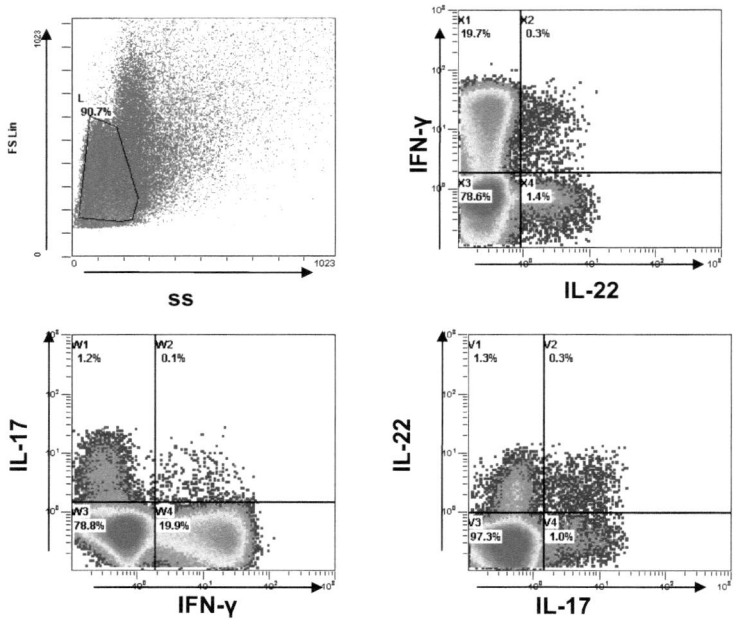

Figure 11 Flow cytometric analysis of IFN-γ, IL-17 and IL-22 in naïve T cells stimulated with 0.03μM FICZ and 10 ng/ml IL-1β, 20 ng/ml IL-6, 10 ng/ml IL-23, 1 ng/ml TGF-β together with anti-CD3 and anti-CD28 mAb.

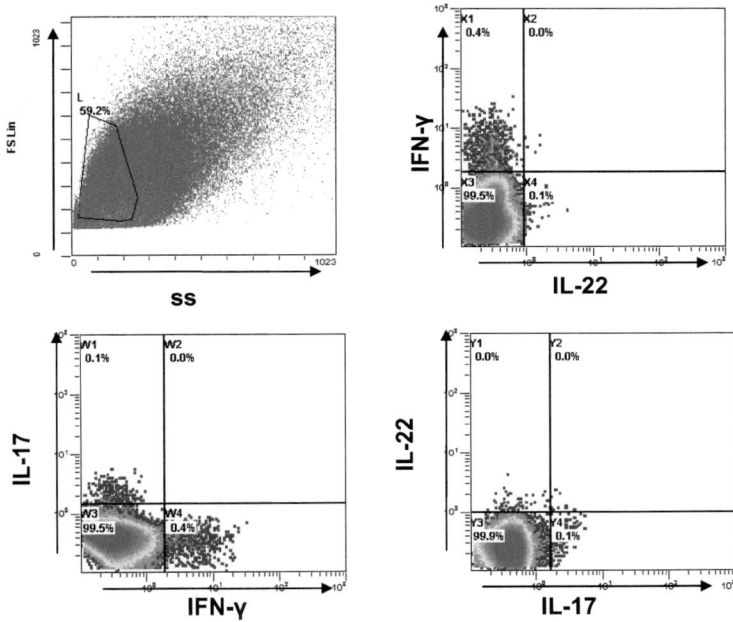

Figure 12 Flow cytometric analysis of IFN-γ, IL-17 and IL-22 in naïve T cells stimulated with 0.03μM FICZ plus 0.03μM TP and 10 ng/ml IL-1β, 20 ng/ml IL-6, 10 ng/ml IL-23, 1 ng/ml TGF-β together with anti-CD3 and anti-CD28 mAb.

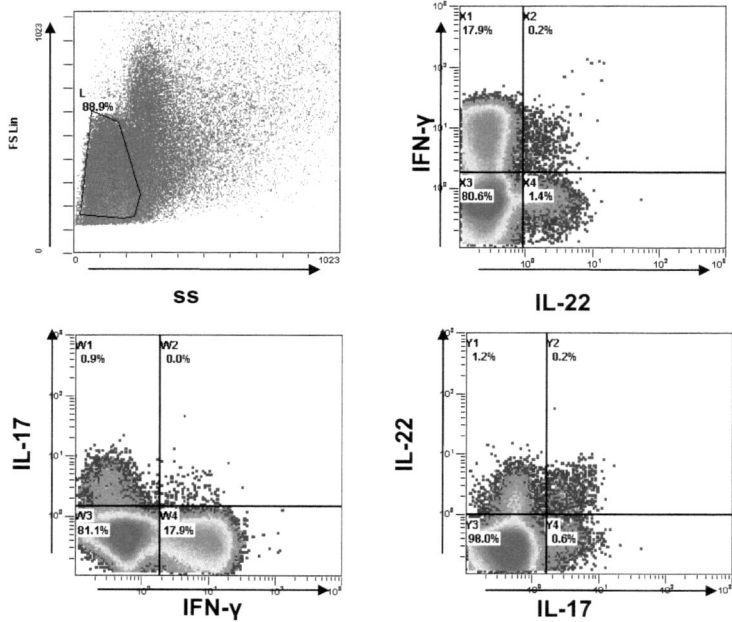

Figure 13 Flow cytometric analysis of IFN-γ, IL-17 and IL-22 in naïve T cells stimulated with 0.03μM FICZ plus 0.003μM TP and 10 ng/ml IL-1β, 20 ng/ml IL-6, 10 ng/ml IL-23, 1 ng/ml TGF-β together with anti-CD3 and anti-CD28 mAb.

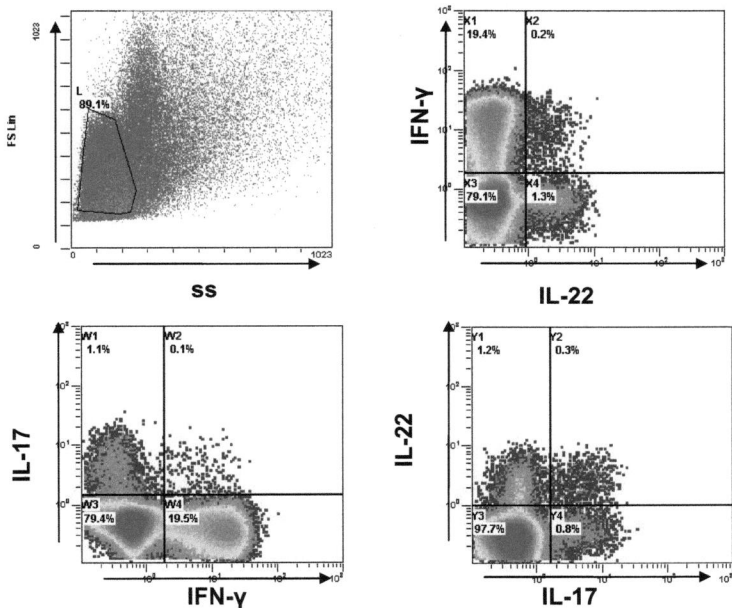

Figure 14 Flow cytometric analysis of IFN-γ, IL-17 and IL-22 in naïve T cells stimulated with 0.03μM FICZ plus 0.0003μM TP and 10 ng/ml IL-1β, 20 ng/ml IL-6, 10 ng/ml IL-23, 1 ng/ml TGF-β together with anti-CD3 and anti-CD28 mAb.

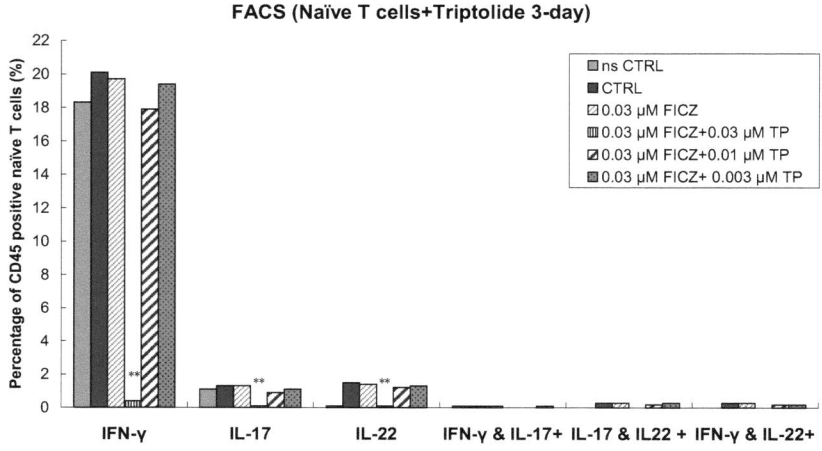

Figure 15 Treatment with triptolide decreased IFN-γ, IL-17 and IL-22 levels and showed a dose-dependent repression of FICZ-induced cytokine expression. nsCTRL, naïve T cells treated with only anti-CD3 and anti-CD28; CTRL, naïve T cells treated with IL-1β, IL-6 and IL-23 together with anti-CD3 and anti-CD28. **P<0.01.

3.5 Apo2.7 cytotoxicity test in naïve T cells

To explore if TP induced apoptosis naïve T cells were treated from the beginning with TP at final concentrations of 0.3μM, 0.1μM, 0.06μM, 0.03μM and 0.01μM. The cells were restimulated with PDBU, ionomycin and brefaldin A after 24h-incubation. Cells were incubated with Apo2.7 antibodies and analyzed by flow cytometric analysis. TP in concentration above 0.03μM induced a significant increase in apoptosis in naïve T cells (Figure 16).

Gated on CD45+ cells example

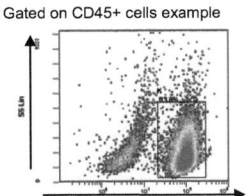

1*10⁶ Naive CD4+ in 1 ml control

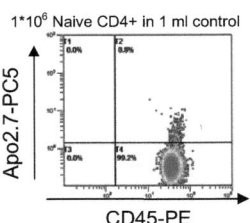

1*10⁶ Naive CD4+ in 1ml 0.3 μM Triptolide

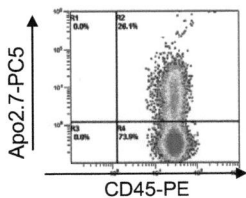

1*10⁶ Naive CD4+ in 1ml 0.1 μM Triptolide

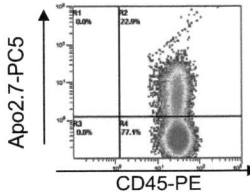

1*10⁶ Naive CD4+ in 1ml 0.06 μM Triptolide

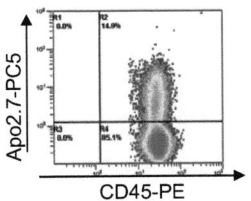

1*10⁶ Naive CD4+ in 1ml 0.03 μM Triptolide

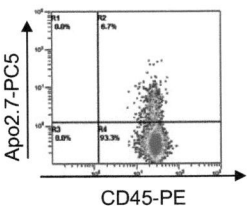

1*10⁶ Naive CD4+ in 1ml 0.01 μM Triptolide

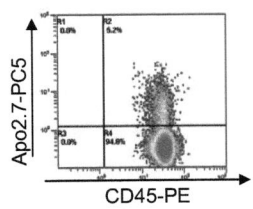

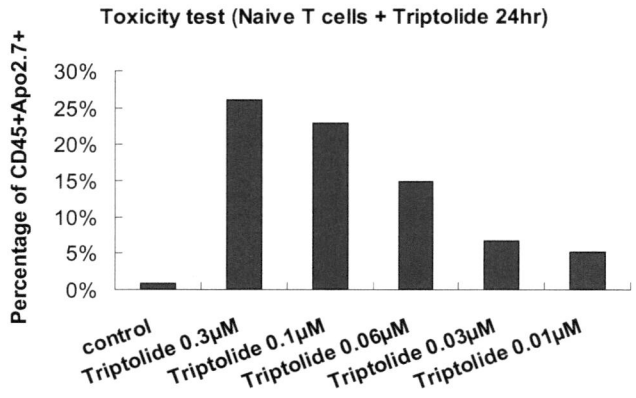

Figure 16 Induction of apoptosis in naïve T cells by triptolide. Expression of the early apoptosis marker Apo2.7 was analyzed by flow cytometry.

3.6 ELISA

To determine whether IFN-γ, IL-17 and IL-22 production was regulated simultaneously at the protein level naïve T cells were incubated with FICZ (0.5μM) alone, FICZ (0.03μM) together with TP (0.03μM) or FICZ (0.03μM) together with various concentrations of TP (0.03, 0.01 to 0.003μM). As shown in Figure 17A, stimulation with FICZ resulted in a high level production of IFN-γ, IL-17 and IL-22 after 72h-incubation. Treatment with TP decreased IFN-γ, IL-17 and IL-22 levels and showed a dose-dependent decrease of FICZ-induced cytokines production.

In a second set of experiments the culture medium was removed after 72h-incubation and naïve T cells were restimulated with PDBU and ionomycin. The supernatants were harvested for ELISA after 5h-incubation. The data are shown in Figure 17B. Stimulation with FICZ resulted in significantly higher levels of IFN-γ, IL-17 and IL-22 as compared to control cultures. When cells were incubated in the presence of various concentrations of TP the production of FICZ-induced IFN-γ, IL-17 and IL-22 was significantly decreased in a dose-dependent manner ($P<0.001$ or $P<0.05$, compared to cultures with FICZ 0.03 μM).

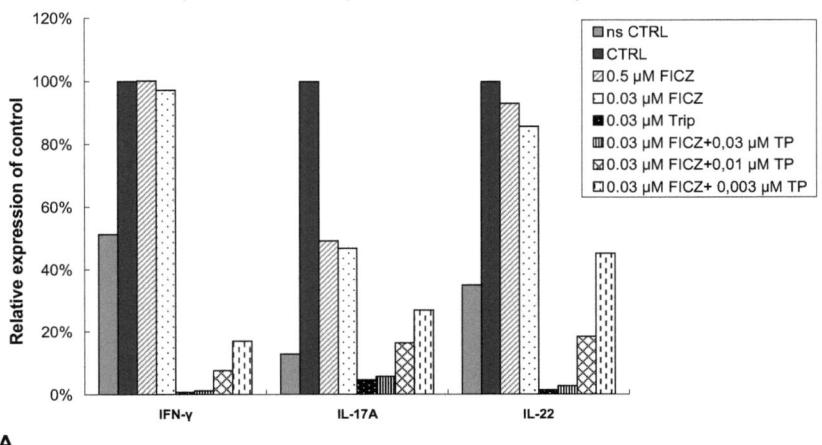

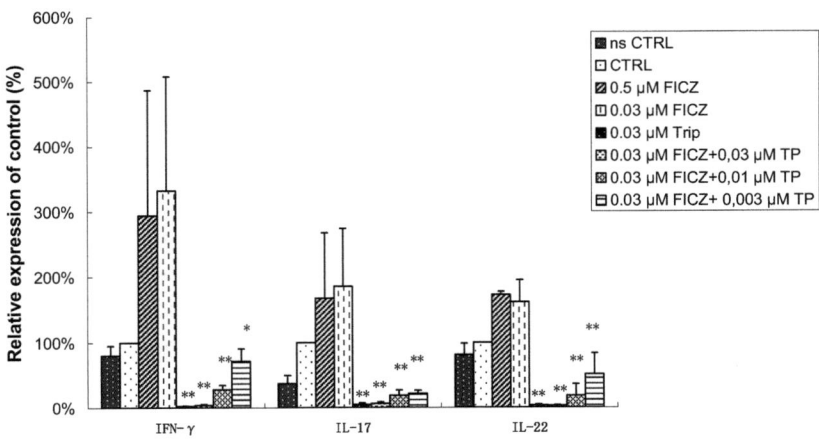

Figure 17 The inhibitory effect of TP on the production of IFN-γ, IL-17 and IL-22 by naïve T cells at the protein level. **(A)** Supernatants were harvested for ELISA after 72h-incubation. **(B)** Naïve T cells were restimulated with PDBU and ionomycin after 72h-incubation. Supernatants were harvested for ELISA after 5h-incubation. nsCTRL, naïve T cells treated with only anti-CD3 and anti-CD28; CTRL, naïve T cells treated with IL-1β, IL-6 and IL-23 together with anti-CD3 and anti-CD28. Mean + SD of three independent experiments. **$P<0.01$.* $P<0.05$.

4. Discussion

Activation of the AhR stimulates T cells to express mRNA and to secrete a range of pro-inflammatory cytokines which contributes to specific activation of the immune system. It is widely accepted that the majority of the transcriptional activity associated with AhR is a consequence of direct agonist binding despite published accounts of AhR activity through loss of cell-cell contact without exogenously added ligand (Cho et al., 2004;Monk et al., 2001) or via indirect activators such as omeprazole (Backlund and Ingelman-Sundberg, 2005). Extended research related to the possible role of AhR biology in inflammation and adaptive immunity (De Souza et al., 2009;Esser et al., 2009;Patel et al., 2009;Veldhoen et al., 2009), raised the notion that inhibition of AhR activity may have therapeutic potential. Thus far, little is known about the molecular mechanism of how AhR is involved in immune regulation. It has been reported that AhR activated by ligands such as TCDD regulates the generation of Tregs and modulates Th1/Th2 balance (Funatake et al., 2005;Negishi, Kato, Ooneda, Mimura, Takada, Mochizuki, Yamamoto, Fujii-Kuriyama, and Furusako, 2005). However, recent evidence has shown that AhR enhances Th17 differentiation and its ligation is essential for induction of IL-22 (Veldhoen et al., 2008). 6-formylindolo[3,2-b]carbazole (FICZ), a tryptophan-derived photoproduct, is thought to be an endogenous agonist with high affinity for the AhR receptor, comparable to TCDD (Nguyen and Bradfield, 2008). Ligation of AhR by FICZ upregulates the expression of IL-17A, IL-17F and IL-22 in human Th17 cells, as well as induction of genes encoding xenobiotic metabolizing cytochrome P450 enzymes such as CYP1A1 and CYP1B1. AhR antagonists reduce Th17 differentiation in naive $CD4^+$ T cells to levels equivalent to those observed for $CD4^+$ T cells from AhR-deficient mice (Jeon and Esser, 2000). Because Th17 cells are the driving force for autoimmune diseases such as inflammatory bowel disease, rheumatoid arthritis, multiple sclerosis and psoriasis it seems possible that AhR-activation exacerbates Th17-mediated autoimmunity. The molecular mechanisms involved in AhR-modulation of the Th17 program are currently not well defined. AhR agonists have been shown to repress or transactivate NF-kB response genes (Zordoky and El Kadi, 2009). It was recently suggested that AhR interacts with STAT1 and STAT5 and that it may regulate Th17 development by modifying the activation of these two negative regulators of Th17 generation (Kimura et al., 2008).

Triptolide has been demonstrated to be effective for the treatment of several autoimmune diseases in both animals and humans (Pan, 1987;Tao et al., 1987). The immunosuppressive effects of TP can be partially attributed to its inhibitory effects on the production of Th1-type cytokines, but not Th2-type cytokines (Tao et al., 1996;Wu et al., 2003b). A recent report showed that triptolide inhibited the differentiation of murine $CD4^+$ T cells into Th17 cells and IL-17 mRNA expression in vitro (Wang et al., 2008b).

In this study we demonstrated for the first time that TP mediates at least part of its in vitro effects via an inhibition of AhR-activation. We were able to show that TP had a suppressive effect on Th17 differentiation in human memory T cells and the ability to inhibit effects induced by the AhR-agonist FICZ thereby deactivating the AhR signaling pathway in both keratinocytes and naive T cells.

With the methods employed (ELISA and flow cytometry) the inhibitiory effect of TP on the biological function of Th1 and Th17 cells was assessed. Consistent with previous reports, TP inhibited anti-CD3/anti-CD28 mAbs stimulated IFN-γ production in human T cells in a dose-dependent manner. In addition, our data confirmed that the presence of IL-1β, IL-6, IL-23 and TGF-β induced an increasing proportion of Th17 cells differentiating from human naïve T cells (Stockinger, Veldhoen, and Martin, 2007;Veldhoen et al., 2008). However, the proportion of Th17 cells generated from human naïve T cells was not so apparent compared to the effect in naïve T cells from mice.

In this study it could be shown that exposure of naive T cells to FICZ substantially enhanced Th17 polarization and induced IL-22 production. TP inhibited the production of IL-17 and IL-22 by more than 95% at a concentration of 0.03μM. The exposure to both FICZ and TP at the same concentration of 0.03μM decreased the production of IL-17 and IL-22 by about 90% indicating that TP may bind to AhR with a higher affinity than FICZ. Moreover, the inhibition of IL-17 and IL-22 production was demonstrated after preincubation and subsequent removal of TP from the culture medium before FICZ-stimulation. These data suggest that the addition of TP during Th17 polarization effectively and directly suppressed differentiation of Th17 cells in vitro. According to the results obtained by FACS-analysis, TP exhibited an inhibitory effect on FICZ-induced production of IL-17 and IL-22 by memory Th17 cells while having no impact on the viability of cells. Unlike CH-223191, the first reported ligand-selective antagonist of AhR (Zhao et al., 2010), TP significantly modulated the differentiation of Th1 cells (Kim et al., 2006).

Employing the method of qPCR we showed that TP significantly inhibited IFN-γ, IL-17 and IL-22 mRNA expression in purified human naive T cells, which is consistent with previously reported data obtained in mice (Wang, Jia, and Wu, 2008). In addition, we showed for the first time that TP potently down-regulated FICZ-induced CYP1A1 and CYP1B1 mRNA expression in both keratinocytes and naive T cells. The transcriptional induction of CYP1A1 and CYP1B1 enzyme isoforms is the best characterized molecular response to AhR activation (Mimura and Fujii-Kuriyama, 2003). Several studies have suggested that chronically expressed cytochrome P450 contributes to TCDD-induced toxicity (Matsumura, 2003;Smith et al., 2001;Uno et al., 2004). This enzyme catalyzes the epoxidation of certain classes of xenobiotics resulting in the generation of highly reactive electrophilic metabolites that may result in genotoxicity. This activity also generates NADH-dependent oxygen radicals, which may lead to indiscriminate damage to cellular macromolecules and ultimately in toxicity (Mandal, 2005;Matsumura, 2003). TP inhibited the FICZ-induced CYP1A1 and CYP1B1 mRNA-expression in a concentration-depend manner indicating that TP inhibited FICZ-mediated cytochrome P450 induction by transcriptional regulation. Therefore, the suppressive effect of TP on IL-17 and IL-22 gene transcription might be related to the inhibition of endogenous AhR activity.

Interestingly, TP revealed no species dependency across the AhR target genes examined, which is also in contrast to previously described antagonists (Zhang et al., 2003). The reason for the variability observed with other reported antagonists is not known but may result from the differences in the rate of uptake, metabolism, intrinsic variation in binding affinity for the AhR or reflect differences in how AhR activity is investigated (Wang and Hankinson, 2002;Zhou and Gasiewicz, 2003).

TP has been shown to induce cell death in a concentration dependend fashion. According to the results of neutral red and MTT assays, TP at the concentration of 0.05µM has no cytostatic effect on keratinocytes. Induction of the early apoptosis marker Apo2.7 as measured by FACS analysis occurred at a TP exposure above 0.03µM in naive T cells. This would imply that the suppressive effect of TP on CYPs transcription and Th17 differentiation might not be related to cytotoxicity. However, this preliminary evidence that TP is non-toxic is limited and restricted to short-term outcomes.

For potential medical application of chemopreventive agents, their safety assessment through many toxicity studies have to be performed, and a full understanding of pharmacokinetics must be achieved. The study about safety and pharmacokinetics of TP deserve further detailed investigation.

In conclusion, we have demonstrated for the first time that the small natural occuring molecule triptolide is a potent AhR antagonist. Furthermore, TP exhibited a high capacity to effectively compete with the established AhR agonist FICZ by inhibiting AhR-mediated gene expression and protein secretion. The inhibitory mode of TP remains to be fully determined. Importantly, TP treatment of keratinocytes and naïve T cells revealed no species dependency with regard to antagonism. Thus, TP represents a very potent antagonist of AhR with limited cytotoxicity and its activity as an AhR-antagonist may be linked to its anti-inflammatory and immune-suppressive effects. Since TP is successfully used as a therapeutic regimen of autoimmune disorders in China, our identification of TP as an AhR-antagonist suggests that the AhR could be a therapeutic target of interest.

5. Summary

In China extracts of the herb Tripterygium wilfordii Hook F. (TwHF) are successfully used to treat psoriasis and other autoimmune and/or inflammatory diseases due to its favorable cost-benefit ratio. Triptolide has turned out to be the active substance of TwHF-extracts and has been shown to exert potent anti-inflammatory and immune-suppressive effects *in vitro* and *in vivo* .

The immunosuppressive action of triptolide has been generally attributed to suppression of T-lymphocyte activation. Recently, it was found that triptolide inhibited the differentiation of murine $CD4^+$ T cells into Th17 cells and decreased the transcription level of interleukin (IL)-17 mRNA and IL-6-induced phosphorylation of STAT3, a key signaling molecule involved in the development of Th17 cells.

The aryl hydrocarbon receptor (AhR) is a ligand-dependent transcription factor best known for mediating the toxicity of dioxin. It was shown that in a $CD4^+$ T-cell lineage of mice AhR expression is restricted to the Th17 cell subset and its ligation results in the production of the Th17 cytokines IL-17 and IL-22. Ligation of AhR by 6-formylindolo[3,2-b]carbazole (FICZ), a tryptophan-derived photoproduct that is thought to be an endogenous agonist with high affinity for the AhR receptor, upregulates the expression of IL-17A, IL-17F and IL-22 in human Th17 cells, as well as induction of genes encoding for the xenobiotic metabolizing cytochrome P450 enzymes such as CYP1A1 and CYP1B1.

From the molecular structure of triptolide the hypothesis was generated that the compound could bind to AhR and serve as either agonist or antagonist. For this purpose it was investigated whether triptolide could induce cell death and if the exposure to triptolide could affect the differentiation of naïve human T cells to Th17 cells and FICZ induced CYP1A1 and CYP1B1 transcription in both keratinocytes and naive T cells.

The results showed that, comparison of Th17 differentiation in naïve T cells by intracellular staining and ELISA after the addition of FICZ together with different concentrations of triptolide showed strongly decreased IFN-γ, IL-17A and IL-22 production in a dose-dependent manner.

Quantitive PCR demonstrated a significant down-regulation of IFN-γ, IL-17A and IL-22 mRNA expression by triptolide in naive T cells. Additionally, triptolide potently down-regulated FICZ-induced CYP1A1 and CYP1B1 mRNA expression in both keratinocytes and naive T cells, which indicates that TP inhibits FICZ-mediated cytochrome P450 induction by transcriptional regulation.

In conclusion, triptolide exhibits a high capacity to effectively compete with AhR agonist thus repressing AhR-mediated gene induction and protein expression, and its treatment of various cell-types reveals no species dependency with regard to antagonism. These data suggest that the activity of triptolide as an AhR-antagonist may be linked to its anti-inflammatory and immune-suppressive effects. Since triptolide is successfully used as a therapeutic of autoimmune disorders in China our identification of triptolide as an AhR-antagonist suggests that the AhR could be a therapeutic target of interest.

6. Reference

Asano K, Matsuishi J, Yu Y, Kasahara T, and Hisamitsu T (1998): Suppressive effects of Tripterygium wilfordii Hook f., a traditional Chinese medicine, on collagen arthritis in mice. Immunopharmacology 39:117-126.

Astroff B, Zacharewski T, Safe S, Arlotto MP, Parkinson A, Thomas P, and Levin W (1988): 6-Methyl-1,3,8-trichlorodibenzofuran as a 2,3,7,8-tetrachlorodibenzo-p-dioxin antagonist: inhibition of the induction of rat cytochrome P-450 isozymes and related monooxygenase activities. Mol Pharmacol 33:231-236.

Backlund M and Ingelman-Sundberg M (2005): Regulation of aryl hydrocarbon receptor signal transduction by protein tyrosine kinases. Cell Signal 17:39-48.

Beischlag TV, Luis MJ, Hollingshead BD, and Perdew GH (2008): The aryl hydrocarbon receptor complex and the control of gene expression. Crit Rev Eukaryot Gene Expr 18:207-250.

Bettelli E, Korn T, and Kuchroo VK (2007): Th17: the third member of the effector T cell trilogy. Curr Opin Immunol 19:652-657.

Boeck G (2001): Current status of flow cytometry in cell and molecular biology, in International Review of Cytology pp 239-298, Academic Press.

Boniface K, Bak-Jensen KS, Li Y, Blumenschein WM, McGeachy MJ, McClanahan TK, McKenzie BS, Kastelein RA, Cua DJ, and de Waal MR (2009): Prostaglandin E2 regulates Th17 cell differentiation and function through cyclic AMP and EP2/EP4 receptor signaling. J Exp Med 206:535-548.

Borenfreund E and Puerner JA (1985a): Toxicity determined in vitro by morphological alterations and neutral red absorption. Toxicol Lett 24:119-124.

Borenfreund E and Puerner JA (1985b): A simple quantitative procedure using monolayer cultures for cytotoxicity assays (HTD/NR-90). J Tissue Cult Meth 9:7-9.

Bradshaw TD and Bell DR (2009): Relevance of the aryl hydrocarbon receptor (AhR) for clinical toxicology. Clin Toxicol (Phila): 47:632-642.

Chan MA, Kohlmeier JE, Branden M, Jung M, and Benedict SH (1999): Triptolide is more effective in preventing T cell proliferation and interferon-gamma production than is FK506. Phytother Res 13:464-467.

Chang DM, Chang WY, Kuo SY, and Chang ML (1997): The effects of traditional antirheumatic herbal medicines on immune response cells. J Rheumatol 24:436-441.

Chang ML, Yang LL, Chang DM, Kuo SY, and Chu SJ (1993): The influence of Chinese traditional medicine on the production and activity of interleukin 1 (IL-1) [in chinese]. Zhonghua Min Guo Wei Sheng Wu Ji Mian Yi Xue Za Zhi 26:15-24.

Chen BJ (2001): Triptolide, a novel immunosuppressive and anti-inflammatory agent purified from a Chinese herb Tripterygium wilfordii Hook F. Leuk Lymphoma 42:253-265.

Chen BJ, Chen Y, Cui X, Fidler JM, and Chao NJ (2002): Mechanisms of tolerance induced by PG490-88 in a bone marrow transplantation model. Transplantation 73:115-121.

Chizzolini C, Chicheportiche R, Alvarez M, de Rham C, Roux-Lombard P, Ferrari-Lacraz S, and Dayer JM (2008): Prostaglandin E2 synergistically with interleukin-23 favors human Th17 expansion. Blood 112:3696-3703.

Cho YC, Zheng W, and Jefcoate CR (2004): Disruption of cell-cell contact maximally but transiently activates AhR-mediated transcription in 10T1/2 fibroblasts. Toxicol Appl Pharmacol 199:220-238.

Cohen JJ, Duke RC, Fadok VA, and Sellins KS (1992): Apoptosis and programmed cell death in immunity. Annu Rev Immunol 10:267-293.

Cooper AM (2007): IL-23 and IL-17 have a multi-faceted largely negative role in fungal infection. Eur J Immunol 37:2680-2682.

De Souza VR, Cabrera WK, Galvan A, Ribeiro OG, De Franco M, Vorraro F, Starobinas N, Massa S, Dragani TA, and Ibanez OM (2009): Aryl hydrocarbon receptor polymorphism modulates DMBA-induced inflammation and carcinogenesis in phenotypically selected mice. Int J Cancer 124:1478-1482.

Denison MS and Nagy SR (2003): Activation of the aryl hydrocarbon receptor by structurally diverse exogenous and endogenous chemicals. Annu Rev Pharmacol Toxicol 43:309-334.

Dubelaar G.B.J. and Gerritzen P.L. (2000): CytoBuoy: a step forward towards using flow cytometry in operational oceanography. Scientia Marina 64:255-265.

Ellis RE, Yuan JY, and Horvitz HR (1991): Mechanisms and functions of cell death. Annu Rev Cell Biol 7:663-698.

Esser C, Rannug A, and Stockinger B (2009): The aryl hydrocarbon receptor in immunity. Trends Immunol 30:447-454.

Funatake CJ, Marshall NB, Steppan LB, Mourich DV, and Kerkvliet NI (2005): Cutting edge: activation of the aryl hydrocarbon receptor by 2,3,7,8-tetrachlorodibenzo-p-dioxin generates a population of CD4+ CD25+ cells with characteristics of regulatory T cells. J Immunol 175:4184-4188.

Gabriel H and Kindermann W (1995): Flow cytometry. Principles and applications in exercise immunology. Sports Med 20:302-320.

Gerbal-Chaloin S, Pichard-Garcia L, Fabre JM, Sa-Cunha A, Poellinger L, Maurel P, and Daujat-Chavanieu M (2006): Role of CYP3A4 in the regulation of the aryl hydrocarbon receptor by omeprazole sulphide. Cell Signal 18:740-750.

Gutian Hospital and Beisha Hospital FP (1972): Report on the therapeutic effect of the herbal medicine Tripterygium wilfordii Hook f on reactive status of leprosy [in Chinese]. Pi Fu Bing Fang Zhi Tong Xun 29-30.

Harrington LE, Hatton RD, Mangan PR, Turner H, Murphy TL, Murphy KM, and Weaver CT (2005): Interleukin 17-producing CD4+ effector T cells develop via a lineage distinct from the T helper type 1 and 2 lineages. Nat Immunol 6:1123-1132.

Harris M, Zacharewski T, Astroff B, and Safe S (1989): Partial antagonism of 2,3,7,8-tetrachlorodibenzo-p-dioxin-mediated induction of aryl hydrocarbon hydroxylase by 6-methyl-1,3,8-trichlorodibenzofuran: mechanistic studies. Mol Pharmacol 35:729-735.

Ho LJ, Chang DM, Chang ML, Kuo SY, and Lai JH (1999): Mechanism of immunosuppression of the antirheumatic herb TWHf in human T cells. J Rheumatol 26:14-24.

Jeon MS and Esser C (2000): The murine IL-2 promoter contains distal regulatory elements responsive to the Ah receptor, a member of the evolutionarily conserved bHLH-PAS transcription factor family. J Immunol 165:6975-6983.

Jiang XH, Wong BC, Lin MC, Zhu GH, Kung HF, Jiang SH, Yang D, and Lam SK (2001): Functional p53 is required for triptolide-induced apoptosis and AP-1 and nuclear factor-kappaB activation in gastric cancer cells. Oncogene 20:8009-8018.

Kim SH, Henry EC, Kim DK, Kim YH, Shin KJ, Han MS, Lee TG, Kang JK, Gasiewicz TA, Ryu SH, and Suh PG (2006): Novel compound 2-methyl-2H-pyrazole-3-carboxylic acid (2-methyl-4-o-tolylazo-phenyl)-amide (CH-223191) prevents 2,3,7,8-TCDD-induced toxicity by antagonizing the aryl hydrocarbon receptor. Mol Pharmacol 69:1871-1878.

Kimura A, Naka T, Nohara K, Fujii-Kuriyama Y, and Kishimoto T (2008): Aryl hydrocarbon receptor regulates STAT1 activation and participates in the development of Th17 cells. Proc Natl Acad Sci U.S.A 105:9721-9726.

Koester SK, Roth P, Mikulka WR, Schlossman SF, Zhang C, and Bolton WE (1997): Monitoring early cellular responses in apoptosis is aided by the mitochondrial membrane protein-specific monoclonal antibody APO2.7. Cytometry 29:306-312.

Kolls JK and Linden A (2004): Interleukin-17 family members and inflammation. Immunity 21:467-476.

Korn T, Oukka M, Kuchroo V, and Bettelli E (2007): Th17 cells: effector T cells with inflammatory properties. Semin Immunol 19:362-371.

Kupchan SM, Court WA, Dailey RG, Jr., Gilmore CJ, and Bryan RF (1972): Triptolide and tripdiolide, novel antileukemic diterpenoid triepoxides from Tripterygium wilfordii. J Am Chem Soc 94:7194-7195.

Laurence A, Tato CM, Davidson TS, Kanno Y, Chen Z, Yao Z, Blank RB, Meylan F, Siegel R, Hennighausen L, Shevach EM, and O'shea JJ (2007): Interleukin-2 signaling via STAT5 constrains T helper 17 cell generation. Immunity 26:371-381.

Liang SC, Tan XY, Luxenberg DP, Karim R, Dunussi-Joannopoulos K, Collins M, and Fouser LA (2006): Interleukin (IL)-22 and IL-17 are coexpressed by Th17 cells and cooperatively enhance expression of antimicrobial peptides. J Exp Med 203:2271-2279.

Liu Q, Chen T, Chen H, Zhang M, Li N, Lu Z, Ma P, and Cao X (2004): Triptolide (PG-490) induces apoptosis of dendritic cells through sequential p38 MAP kinase phosphorylation and caspase 3 activation. Biochem Biophys Res Commun 319:980-986.

Lümann-Rauch R (1979): Drug-induced lysosomal storage disorders., in Lysosomes in applied biology and therapeutics (J.T.Dingle, P.J.Jacques, and I.H.Shaw eds). North-Holland Publishing Co., Amsterdam.

Lowes MA, Bowcock AM, and Krueger JG (2007): Pathogenesis and therapy of psoriasis. Nature 445:866-873.

Lu YF, Santostefano M, Cunningham BD, Threadgill MD, and Safe S (1995): Identification of 3'-methoxy-4'-nitroflavone as a pure aryl hydrocarbon (Ah) receptor antagonist and evidence for more than one form of the nuclear Ah receptor in MCF-7 human breast cancer cells. Arch Biochem Biophys 316:470-477.

Luster MI, Hong LH, Osborne R, Blank JA, Clark G, Silver MT, Boorman GA, and Greenlee WF (1986): 1-amino-3,7,8-trichlorodibenzo-p-dioxin: a specific antagonist for TCDD-induced myelotoxicity. Biochem Biophys Res Commun 139:747-756.

Mandal PK (2005): Dioxin: a review of its environmental effects and its aryl hydrocarbon receptor biology. J Comp Physiol B 175:221-230.

Matsumura F (2003): On the significance of the role of cellular stress response reactions in the toxic actions of dioxin. Biochem Pharmacol 66:527-540.

Michael C.Alley, Dominic A.Scudiero, Anne Monks, and Miriam L.Hursey (1988): Feasibility of Drug Screening with Panels of Human Tumor Cell Lines Using a Microculture Tetrazolium Assay. Cancer Res 589-601.

Mimura J and Fujii-Kuriyama Y (2003): Functional role of AhR in the expression of toxic effects by TCDD. Biochim Biophys Acta 1619:263-268.

Monk SA, Denison MS, and Rice RH (2001): Transient expression of CYP1A1 in rat epithelial cells cultured in suspension. Arch Biochem Biophys 393:154-162.

Mrowietz U, Kragballe K, Reich K, Spuls P, Griffiths CE, Nast A, Franke J, Antoniou C, Arenberger P, Balieva F, Bylaite M, Correia O, Daudén E, Gisondi P, Iversen L, Kemény L, Lahfa M, Nijsten T, Rantanen T, Reich A, Rosenbach T, Segaert S, Smith C, Talme T, Volc-Platzer B, Yawalkar N (2011): Definition of treatment goals for moderate to severe psoriasis: a European consensus. Arch Dermatol Res 303:1-11.

Mucida D, Park Y, Kim G, Turovskaya O, Scott I, Kronenberg M, and Cheroutre H (2007): Reciprocal TH17 and regulatory T cell differentiation mediated by retinoic acid. Science 317:256-260.

Murray IA, Flaveny CA, DiNatale BC, Chairo CR, Schroeder JC, Kusnadi A, and Perdew GH (2010): Antagonism of aryl hydrocarbon receptor signaling by 6,2',4'-trimethoxyflavone. J Pharmacol Exp Ther 332:135-144.

Napolitani G, Acosta-Rodriguez EV, Lanzavecchia A, and Sallusto F (2009): Prostaglandin E2 enhances Th17 responses via modulation of IL-17 and IFN-gamma production by memory CD4+ T cells. Eur J Immunol 39:1301-1312.

Nast A, Kopp I, Augustin M, Banditt KB, Boehncke WH, Follmann M, Friedrich M, Huber M, Kahl C, Klaus J, Koza J, Kreiselmaier I, Mohr J, Mrowietz U, Ockenfels HM, Orzechowski HD, Prinz J, Reich K, Rosenbach T, Rosumeck S, Schlaeger M, Schmid-Ott G, Sebastian M, Streit V, Weberschock T, and Rzany B (2007): German evidence-based guidelines for the treatment of Psoriasis vulgaris (short version). Arch Dermatol Res 299:111-138.

Nebert DW and Karp CL (2008): Endogenous functions of the aryl hydrocarbon receptor (AHR): intersection of cytochrome P450 1 (CYP1)-metabolized eicosanoids and AHR biology. J Biol Chem 283:36061-36065.

Negishi T, Kato Y, Ooneda O, Mimura J, Takada T, Mochizuki H, Yamamoto M, Fujii-Kuriyama Y, and Furusako S (2005): Effects of aryl hydrocarbon receptor signaling on the modulation of TH1/TH2 balance. J Immunol 175:7348-7356.

Nguyen LP and Bradfield CA (2008): The search for endogenous activators of the aryl hydrocarbon receptor. Chem Res Toxicol. 21:102-116.

Nicholson DW (1996): ICE/CED3-like proteases as therapeutic targets for the control of inappropriate apoptosis. Nat Biotechnol 14:297-301.

Nurieva R, Yang XO, Martinez G, Zhang Y, Panopoulos AD, Ma L, Schluns K, Tian Q, Watowich SS, Jetten AM, and Dong C (2007): Essential autocrine regulation by IL-21 in the generation of inflammatory T cells. Nature 448:480-483.

Ohtake F, Fujii-Kuriyama Y, and Kato S (2007): Transcription factor AhR is a ligand-dependent E3 ubiquitin ligase. Tanpakushitsu Kakusan Koso 52:1973-1979.

Okey AB (2007): An aryl hydrocarbon receptor odyssey to the shores of toxicology: the Deichmann Lecture, International Congress of Toxicology-XI. Toxicol Sci 98:5-38.

Pan YR (1987): Treatment of purpura nephritis with Tripterygium wilfordii Hook f [in Chinese]. Acta Acad Med Sin 2-4.

Patel RD, Murray IA, Flaveny CA, Kusnadi A, and Perdew GH (2009): Ah receptor represses acute-phase response gene expression without binding to its cognate response element. Lab Invest 89:695-707.

Pepper C, Thomas A, Tucker H, Hoy T, and Bentley P (1998): Flow cytometric assessment of three different methods for the measurement of in vitro apoptosis. Leuk Res 22:439-444.

Qiu D and Kao PN (2003): Immunosuppressive and anti-inflammatory mechanisms of triptolide, the principal active diterpenoid from the Chinese medicinal herb Tripterygium wilfordii Hook. f. Drugs R D 4:1-18.

Quintana FJ, Basso AS, Iglesias AH, Korn T, Farez MF, Bettelli E, Caccamo M, Oukka M, and Weiner HL (2008): Control of T(reg) and T(H)17 cell differentiation by the aryl hydrocarbon receptor. Nature 453:65-71.

Raychaudhuri SP and Farber EM (2001): The prevalence of psoriasis in the world. J Eur Acad Dermatol Venereol 15:16-17.

Reiners JJ, Jr., Lee JY, Clift RE, Dudley DT, and Myrand SP (1998): PD98059 is an equipotent antagonist of the aryl hydrocarbon receptor and inhibitor of mitogen-activated protein kinase. Mol Pharmacol 53:438-445.

Sambrook J (1989): Molecular cloning a laboratory manual. Cold Spring Harbor Laboratory Press, Cold Spring Harbor, NY.

Savige JA, Paspaliaris B, Silvestrini R, Davies D, Nikoloutsopoulos T, Sturgess A, Neil J, Pollock W, Dunster K, and Hendle M (1998): A review of immunofluorescent patterns associated with antineutrophil cytoplasmic antibodies (ANCA) and their differentiation from other antibodies. J Clin Pathol 51:568-575.

Shapiro HM (2005): Practical Flow Cytometry.

Slater TF, Sawzer B, and Straeuli U (1963): Studies on succinate-tetrazolium reductase system. III. Points of coupling of four different tetrazolium salts, Biochim.Biophys Acta 77:383-393.

Smith AG, Clothier B, Carthew P, Childs NL, Sinclair PR, Nebert DW, and Dalton TP (2001): Protection of the Cyp1a2(-/-) null mouse against uroporphyria and hepatic injury following exposure to 2,3,7,8-tetrachlorodibenzo-p-dioxin. Toxicol Appl Pharmacol 173:89-98.

Stein DS, Korvick JA, and Vermund SH (1992): CD4+ lymphocyte cell enumeration for prediction of clinical course of human immunodeficiency virus disease: a review. J Infect Dis 165:352-363.

Stockinger B, Veldhoen M, and Martin B (2007): Th17 T cells: linking innate and adaptive immunity. Semin Immunol 19:353-361.

Stumhofer JS, Laurence A, Wilson EH, Huang E, Tato CM, Johnson LM, Villarino AV, Huang Q, Yoshimura A, Sehy D, Saris CJ, O'Shea JJ, Hennighausen L, Ernst M, and Hunter CA (2006): Interleukin 27 negatively regulates the development of interleukin 17-producing T helper cells during chronic inflammation of the central nervous system. Nat Immunol 7:937-945.

Tao X, Davis LS, Hashimoto K, and Lipsky PE (1996): The Chinese herbal remedy, T2, inhibits mitogen-induced cytokine gene transcription by T cells, but not initial signal transduction. J Pharmacol Exp Ther 276:316-325.

Tao X, Schulze-Koops H, Ma L, Cai J, Mao Y, and Lipsky PE (1998): Effects of Tripterygium wilfordii hook F extracts on induction of cyclooxygenase 2 activity and prostaglandin E2 production. Arthritis Rheum 41:130-138.

Tao XL, Sun Y, and Dong Y (1987): A double-blind, controlled trial of Tripterygium wilfordii glycosides in the treatment of rheumatoid arthritis. Arthritis Rheum 59.

Tao X and Lipsky PE (2000): The Chinese anti-inflammatory and immunosuppressive herbal remedy Tripterygium wil- fordii Hook F. Complementary and alternative therapies for rheumatic diseases II. Rheumatic Disease Clinics of North America 26:29-50.

Thompson CB (1995): Apoptosis in the pathogenesis and treatment of disease. Science 267:1456-1462.

Tian Y, Rabson AB, and Gallo MA (2002): Ah receptor and NF-kappaB interactions: mechanisms and physiological implications. Chem Biol Interact 141:97-115.

Uno S, Dalton TP, Sinclair PR, Gorman N, Wang B, Smith AG, Miller ML, Shertzer HG, and Nebert DW (2004): Cyp1a1(-/-) male mice: protection against high-dose TCDD-induced lethality and wasting syndrome, and resistance to intrahepatocyte lipid accumulation and uroporphyria. Toxicol Appl Pharmacol 196:410-421.

van de Loosdrecht AA, Beelen RHJ, Ossenkoppele GJ, Broekhoven MG, and Langenhuijsen MMAC (1940): A tetrazolium-based colorimetric MTT assay to quantitate human monocyte mediated cytotoxicity against leukemic cells from cell lines and patients with acute myeloid leukemia. J Immunol Meth 174:311-320.

Veldhoen M, Hirota K, Christensen J, O'Garra A, and Stockinger B (2009): Natural agonists for aryl hydrocarbon receptor in culture medium are essential for optimal differentiation of Th17 T cells. J Exp Med 206:43-49.

Veldhoen M, Hirota K, Westendorf AM, Buer J, Dumoutier L, Renauld JC, and Stockinger B (2008): The aryl hydrocarbon receptor links TH17-cell-mediated autoimmunity to environmental toxins. Nature 453:106-109.

Wang S and Hankinson O (2002): Functional involvement of the Brahma/SWI2-related gene 1 protein in cytochrome P4501A1 transcription mediated by the aryl hydrocarbon receptor complex. J Biol Chem 277:11821-11827.

Wang X, Matta R, Shen G, Nelin LD, Pei D, and Liu Y (2006): Mechanism of triptolide-induced apoptosis: Effect on caspase activation and Bid cleavage and essentiality of the hydroxyl group of triptolide. J Mol Med 84:405-415.

Wang Y, Jia L, and Wu CY (2008): Triptolide inhibits the differentiation of Th17 cells and suppresses collagen-induced arthritis. Scand J Immunol 68:383-390.

Wedemeyer N and Potter T (2001): Flow cytometry: an 'old' tool for novel applications in medical genetics. Clin Genet 60:1-8.

Wei X, Gong J, Zhu J, Wang P, Li N, Zhu W, and Li J (2008): The suppressive effect of triptolide on chronic colitis and TNF-alpha/TNFR2 signal pathway in interleukin-10 deficient mice. Clin Immunol 129:211-218.

Wilhelmsson A, Whitelaw ML, Gustafsson JA, and Poellinger L (1994): Agonistic and antagonistic effects of alpha-naphthoflavone on dioxin receptor function. Role of the basic region helix-loop-helix dioxin receptor partner factor Arnt. J Biol Chem 269:19028-19033.

Wu Y, Wang Y, Zhong C, Li Y, Li X, and Sun B (2003): The suppressive effect of triptolide on experimental autoimmune uveoretinitis by down-regulating Th1-type response. Int Immunopharmacol 3:1457-1465.

Wyllie AH, Kerr JF, and Currie AR (1980): Cell death: the significance of apoptosis. Int Rev Cytol 68:251-306.

Yao Z, Painter SL, Fanslow WC, Ulrich D, Macduff BM, Spriggs MK, and Armitage RJ (1995): Human IL-17: a novel cytokine derived from T cells. J Immunol 155:5483-5486.

Yip SY (1984): The prevalence of psoriasis in the Mongoloid race. J Am Acad Dermatol 10:965-968.

Zhang C, Ao Z, Seth A, and Schlossman SF (1996): A mitochondrial membrane protein defined by a novel monoclonal antibody is preferentially detected in apoptotic cells. J Immunol 157:3980-3987.

Zhang S, Qin C, and Safe SH (2003): Flavonoids as aryl hydrocarbon receptor agonists/antagonists: effects of structure and cell context. Environ Health Perspect 111:1877-1882.

Zhao B, Degroot DE, Hayashi A, He G, and Denison MS (2010): CH223191 is a ligand-selective antagonist of the Ah (Dioxin) receptor. Toxicol Sci 117:393-403.

Zhou J and Gasiewicz TA (2003): 3'-methoxy-4'-nitroflavone, a reported aryl hydrocarbon receptor antagonist, enhances Cyp1a1 transcription by a dioxin responsive element-dependent mechanism. Arch Biochem Biophys 416:68-80.

Zordoky BN and El Kadi AO (2009): Role of NF-kappaB in the regulation of cytochrome P450 enzymes. Curr Drug Metab 10:164-178.

7. Acknowledgements

I want to express my sincere gratitude to my mentor, Prof. Dr. med. Ulrich Mrowietz, for his invitation to Kiel and the great support of my work, for his scientific guidance and careful correction of the thesis and for his encouragement.

Further, I want to thank the director of the Department of Dermatology, University of Kiel, Prof. Dr. med. Thomas Schwarz, for providing me with the laboratory facilities at the institution to conduct the experiments.

I would also like to thank Dr. rer. nat. Martin Rostami Yazdi, Mrs. Ramona Jurgeleit, and Ms. Lisa-Marie Philipp for their kind help to resolve technical problems and their steady support.

I am also deeply indebted to all the other colleagues of mine, both in Kiel and in Hangzhou, who have given me a lot of support for my study and living in Kiel. This is gratefully acknowledged.

I should finally like to express my gratitude to my beloved parents who have always been supporting without a word of complaint.

8. Curriculum Vitae

Surame:	Han
Name:	Rui
Sex:	Female
Date of Birth:	October 13th, 1983
Place of birth:	Shandong, P.R. China
Address:	Department of Dermatology
	University Medical Center of Schleswig-Holstein, Campus Kiel
	Arnold-Heller-Str. 3, Bldg 19
	24105 Kiel, Germany

Education:

1990-1995	Jishu Primary School, Shengli Oil Field, Shandong
1996-1999	No.59 Middle School, Shengli Oil Field, Shandong
1999-2002	No.1 High School, Shengli Oil Field, Shandong
2002-2007	School of Medicine, Zhejiang Medical Univeristy
	Graduated with the Bachelor Degree of medicine
2007-2008	School of Medicine, Julius-Maximilians-Universität Würzburg
	Exchange student
2008-2009	School of Medicine, Zhejiang Medical Univeristy
	Graduate with the Master Degree of medicine
2009 since Sep.	Dept. of Dermatology, University hospital of Christian-Albrechts-University of Kiel

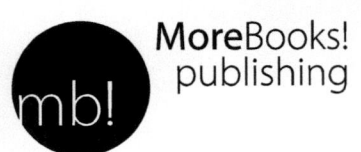
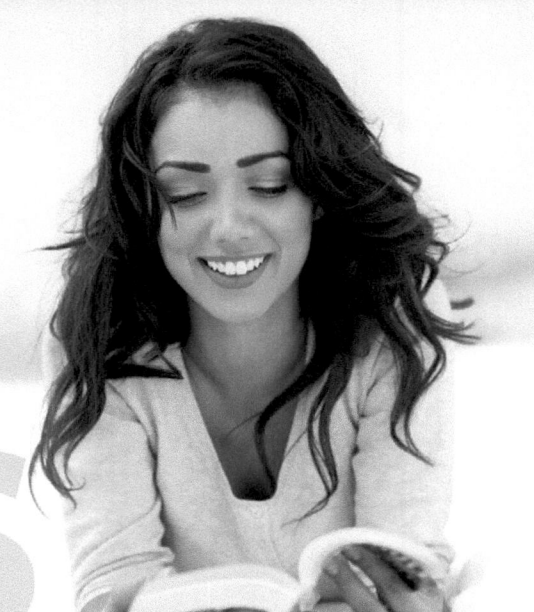

i want morebooks!

Buy your books fast and straightforward online - at one of world's fastest growing online book stores! Environmentally sound due to Print-on-Demand technologies.

Buy your books online at
www.get-morebooks.com

Kaufen Sie Ihre Bücher schnell und unkompliziert online – auf einer der am schnellsten wachsenden Buchhandelsplattformen weltweit! Dank Print-On-Demand umwelt- und ressourcenschonend produziert.

Bücher schneller online kaufen
www.morebooks.de

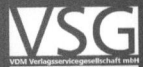 VDM Verlagsservicegesellschaft mbH
Heinrich-Böcking-Str. 6-8   Telefon: +49 681 3720 174   info@vdm-vsg.de
D - 66121 Saarbrücken   Telefax: +49 681 3720 1749   www.vdm-vsg.de

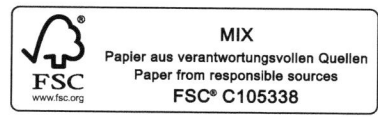

Printed by Books on Demand GmbH, Norderstedt / Germany